Nursing Leaders Speak Out

Issues and Opinions

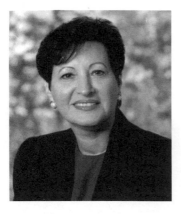

Harriet R. Feldman, PhD, RN, FAAN, is dean and professor at the Lienhard School of Nursing at Pace University. She is also Chairperson of the University's Institutional Review Board. She was one of the founding editors of *Scholarly Inquiry for Nursing Practice* and is currently editor of *Nursing Leadership Forum*, both published by Springer Publishing. Dr. Feldman received her nursing diploma from Long Island College Hospital School of Nursing, bachelor's and master's degrees from Adelphi University, and her PhD from New York University. She also received a certificate for her attendance at the Management Development Program at Harvard University. She has served in leadership positions in a number of local, state, and national professional groups, presented and consulted widely both nationally and internationally, and published extensively in books and refereed journals. Her most recent book, coauthored with Dr. Sandra B. Lewenson is entitled *Nurses in the Political Arena: The Public Face of Nursing* (Springer Publishing) and was named an *American Journal of Nursing* Book-of-the-Year.

Nursing Leaders Speak Out

Issues and Opinions

Harriet R. Feldman, PhD, RN, FAAN
Editor

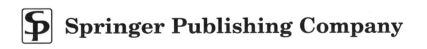 **Springer Publishing Company**

Springer Publishing Company, Inc.
536 Broadway
New York, NY 10012-3955

Acquisitions Editor: *Ruth Chasek*
Production Editor: *Elizabeth Keech*
Cover design by *Susan Hauley*

01 02 03 04 05/5 4 3 2 1

Library of Congress Cataloging-in-Publication Data

Nursing leaders speak out : issues and opinions /
    Harriet R. Feldman, editor.
       p.   ; cm.
    Includes bibliographical references and index.
    ISBN 0-8261-1416-4
       1. Nursing services—Administration.   2. Nurses—Interviews.
    3. Leadership.   I. Feldman, Harriet R.   II. Title: Nursing leadership
    forum.
    [DNLM: 1. Nursing—organization & administration—Collected Works.
    2. Delivery of Health Care—organization & administration—Collected
    Works.   3. Nurse Adminstration—Collected Works.   4. Nursing Care—
    organization & administration—Collected Works.   5. Philosophy, Nursing
    —Collected Works. WY 105 N97474 2001]
    RT42 N864 2001
    362.1'73'068—dc21
                                                              00-069816

Printed in the United States of America by Capital City Press, USA

This book is a compilation of articles previously published in the journal
Nursing Leadership Forum (Springer Publishing Company).

Contents

Contributors   ix

Foreword by Barbara Stevens Barnum   xi

Introduction by Harriet R. Feldman   xiii

Part I: Point/Counterpoint on Contemporary Issues

1. Case Management: Is It Improving Health Outcomes?
    Point: *Dominick L. Flarey*   3
    Counterpoint: *Lucille Lombardi Travis*   7

2. Continuous Quality Improvement: Cult or Science?
    Point: *Janis P. Bellack*   11
    Counterpoint: *Farrokh Alemi*   15

3. Genetics Counseling: Should It Be a Basic Competency
    for Nurses?
    Point: *Constance Visovsky*   23
    Counterpoint: *M. Linda Workman*   28

4. The Shift of Acute Care From the Hospital to the Home:
    Is It a Good Trend?
    Point: *Christine A. Pierce*   33
    Counterpoint: *Bette K. Idemoto*   37

5. Holistic Care: Is It Feasible in Today's Health Care
    Environment?
    Point: *Barbara M. Dossey*   41
    Counterpoint: *Kathy Kolcaba*   49

6. Telehealth: Can Nursing Values Be Preserved?
   Point: *Josette Jones*   55
   Counterpoint: *Shirley M. Moore*   58

7. Building a Better Mousetrap: The Upside of Downsizing
   Education: *Cynthia Caroselli*   63
   Practice: *Joanne Baggerly*   71

8. Sharing the Vision: The Views From Nursing Management and Staff
   Management: *Tara A. Cortes*   77
   Staff: *Cynthia Caroselli*   82

9. Acute Care Nurse Practitioners: An Idea Whose Time Has Come?
   Point: *Joan E. King*   89
   Counterpoint: *Barbara J. Daly*   92

10. Primary and Secondary Prevention: How Much a Part of Nursing?
   Point: *Nancy T. Artinian*   97
   Counterpoint: *Kimberly Adams-Davis*   104

11. Unlicensed Personnel: A Threat to Nursing and Patients?
   Point: *Darlene L. Cox*   109
   Counterpoint: *Mary Jane Kalafut DiMattio*   114

Part II: Interviews With Nursing Leaders

A. Elected and Appointed Public Officials

12. Interview With Imogene King, RN, EdD, FAAN   125
   Sandra B. Lewenson

13. Interview With Diane O. McGivern, RN, PhD, FAAN   137
   Barbara Stevens Barnum

B. Caregivers

14. Interview With Eugene Sawicki, RN, EdD, MDiv, JCL:
   When the Nurse Is a Priest   151
   Barbara Stevens Barnum

15. Interview With Karen Soto, RN, BSN,
and Rosalee Whyte, RN, BSN: The Challenge of
Providing Nursing Care for the Dying   159
Barbara Stevens Barnum

C. Entrepreneur

16. Interview With Carolyn S. Zagury, MS, RN, CPC:
Nurse Entrepreneur and Publisher   173
Barbara Stevens Barnum

D. Educator/Administrator

17. Interview With Marilyn Jaffe-Ruiz, EdD, RN   185
Sandra B. Lewenson

E. Historian

18. Interview With Joan Lynaugh, RN, PhD, FAAN   193
Sandra B. Lewenson

Index   207

Contributors

Kimberly Adams-Davis, ND,
RNC, WhNP, FAAN
Assistant Professor
Frances Payne Bolton School of
Nursing
Case Western Reserve University
Cleveland, Ohio

Farrokh Alemi, PhD
Associate Professor of Health Care
Management
College of Nursing and Health Sciences
George Mason University
Fairfax, Virginia

Nancy T. Artinian, PhD, RN
Associate Professor
College of Nursing
Wayne State University
Detroit, Michigan

Joanne Baggerly, RN, MS,
CRRN, CNRN
Director of Clinical Development
Braintree Hospital Rehabilitation
Network
Braintree, Massachusetts

Barbara Stevens Barnum, PhD,
RN, FAAN
Writer and Consultant
Former Editor, *Nursing Leadership
Forum*
New York, New York

Janis P. Bellack, PhD, RN, FAAN
Associate Provost for Educational
Programs and Professor of Nursing
Medical University of South Carolina
Charleston, South Carolina

Cynthia Caroselli, RN, PhD
Director, Neuroscience and
Restorative Care Center
Mount Sinai Hospital
New York, New York

Tara A. Cortes, PhD, RN, CNAA
Director
Primary Care and Medical Services
Mount Sinai Medical Center
New York, New York

Darlene L. Cox, MS, RN
CEO
East Orange General Hospital
East Orange, New Jersey

Barbara J. Daly, PhD, RN, FAAN
Associate Professor
Frances Payne Bolton School of
Nursing
Case Western Reserve University
Cleveland, Ohio

Barbara M. Dossey, MS, RN,
HNC, FAAN
Director
Holistic Nursing Consultants
Santa Fe, New Mexico

Dominick L. Flarey, PhD, MBA,
RN, CS, CNAA, FACHE
President
Dominick L. Flarey & Associates, Inc.
Niles, Ohio

Bette K. Idemoto, MSN, RN,
CS, CCRN
Department of Vascular Surgery
University Hospitals of Cleveland
Cleveland, Ohio

Josette Jones, RNC, Licentiate
Nursing, Licentiate MIS
Doctoral Candidate
School of Nursing/Industrial
Engineering
University of Wisconsin, Madison
Madison, Wisconsin

Mary Jane Kalafut DiMattio,
MSN, RN
Instructor
Department of Nursing
University of Scranton
Scranton, Pennsylvania

Joan E. King, RN, PhD, ACNP,
ANP
Director, Acute Care Nurse
Practitioner Program
School of Nursing
Vanderbilt University
Nashville, Tennessee

Kathy Kolcaba, PhD, RNC
Assistant Professor
School of Nursing
University of Akron
Akron, Ohio

Sandra B. Lewenson, RN, EdD,
FAAN
Associate Dean and Professor
Lienhard School of Nursing
Pace University
Pleasantville, New York

Shirley M. Moore, RN, PhD
Associate Professor of Nursing
Frances Payne Bolton School of
Nursing
Case Western Reserve University
Cleveland, Ohio

Christine A. Pierce, RN, CS,
MSN, CHCE
Administrative Director
Cleveland Clinic Home Care
Cleveland Clinic Foundation
Valley View, Ohio

Lucille Lombardi Travis, PhD,
RN, CNA
Associate Dean and Associate
Professor
Texas Women's University, Houston
Center
Houston, Texas

Constance Visovsky, RN, MS,
ACNP
Research Project Director/ Acute
Care Nurse Practitioner
Frances Payne Bolton School of
Nursing
Case Western University
Cleveland, Ohio

M. Linda Workman, PhD, RN,
FAAN
Associate Professor
College of Nursing
University of Cincinnati
Cincinnati, Ohio

Foreword

This unique book compiles articles that, in every case, tell us as much about the authors as we learn about the subject matter. The first half of the book, focusing on point/counterpoint, makes those differences stand out, either by giving opposing views, or, alternately, by providing different viewpoints on the same subject matter. In either case, we come away knowing a great deal about an author.

I'm committed to seeing such alternate and opposing visions given voice in nursing. We need to remember that there is no one right answer to any of nursing's problems. Otherwise we'd have solved them all years ago. We also need to struggle against the urge to latch onto a single viewpoint and denigrate all others. Nurses have a tendency to want to do that, perhaps as a way of avoiding conflict. This book, however, serves as a reminder that we should cherish our diversity, not seek to do away with it.

I love nothing more than when an author challenges one of nursing's sacred cows. We see that happen in this book when authors look at both sides of such issues as downsizing or the use of unlicensed personnel. I hope this collection will spur the reader to take one of his/her own sacred cows and look at it afresh. Leadership more often arises from a disparate viewpoint than from a reaffirmation of what is already accepted. Let's encourage diversity in nursing in all its aspects—not simply in transcultural nursing.

The second half of the book continues its focus on individual opinions, this time through the interview process. In most cases, an interview takes on a certain vitality that is lost when an article is carefully worked and reworked. Smooth edges are sacrificed in an interview, but they are compensated for by the drama and intensity that comes across in most people being interviewed. An interview is a great combination of personal feeling and subject matter content. Interviews also reveal how very many differences we find in a group of leaders from the same profession.

Hopefully, then, this book will help the reader celebrate our differences, our unique viewpoints, at the same time giving some really thoughtful approaches to many of our professional dilemmas.

BARBARA STEVENS BARNUM
RN, PHD, FAAN

Introduction

Nursing Leaders Speak Out is an introduction to the views and opinions of distinguished nurses on issues of concern in nursing today. It is derived from the journal *Nursing Leadership Forum*, which has published a Point/Counterpoint column and interviews with nursing leaders since its inception in 1995. In the first instance, experts from opposing sides offer perspectives on innovative ideas, models of care, ethics, and values. In the second, distinguished leaders in nursing and health care help us to better understand nursing's history and impact. Together these writings are fitting examples of a public dialogue that conveys the values and practices of the nursing profession.

The book is divided into two sections. The Point/Counterpoint section reflects the multifaceted nature of contemporary issues. Each issue is discussed from a pro and con standpoint, by nurses with opposing views. The issues discussed include continuous quality improvement, genetics counseling, the shift of acute care from hospital to home, holistic care, telehealth, workplace redesign, the changing role of the nurse in clinical practice, and case management. In the second section, distinguished nurses voice their experiences and opinions in an interview format. Here are examples of some of the dialogues you will encounter in Part I:

On Genetics Counseling
Planned to run through 2003, the Human Genome Project aims to determine the DNA sequence of every gene in the human body. As information is revealed, science and medicine will be transformed. Nurses are in a critical position to ensure accessibility to information, including risks and benefits, and to inter-

act with individuals, families, and communities. What should the role of the nurse be?

Constance Visovsky, RN, MS, ACNP: "Nurses must now be prepared to meet the challenges of incorporating an understanding of this new technology into their everyday practice."

M. Linda Workman, PhD, RN, FAAN: "The issue is not whether nurses *can* perform genetic counseling but rather, *should* they perform genetic counseling, given the minimal genetics preparation available in most basic nursing programs...Giving nurses the responsibility of genetic counseling without providing them with the tools of authority (adequate education) is a recipe for disaster."

On Holistic Care
There is a growing public awareness of the role of alternative therapies in the prevention and treatment of disease. Nurses have been advocating holistic care since the time of Florence Nightingale. Many nursing education programs incorporate concepts of holistic care. What is the feasibility of providing holistic care in today's health care settings?

Barbara Dossey, MS, RN, HNC, FAAN: "A frequently asked question is whether or not holistic care can be delivered in today's health care environment, and the answer is, yes, it can."

Kathy Kolcaba, PhD, RNC: "Some nurses continue to align themselves with the medical model...Should this infatuation continue, holistic care cannot be valued or delivered."

On the Shift of Acute Care From the Hospital to the Home
The home care focus has come full circle, since public health nursing began in the community long before hospitals existed. In shifting from the hospital back to the home, what are the advantages and disadvantages to this movement?

Christine A. Pierce, RN, CS, MSN, CHCE: "The shift of patients to home health care is beneficial from a number of perspectives—not the least of which is avoidance of the inherent risks of an inpatient stay."

Bette K. Idemoto, MSN, RN, CS, CCRN: "The decreased level of funding and subsequent loss of home care assistance upon early discharge may result in increased readmissions and emergency room visits."

On Case Management
The landscape of health care delivery and nursing practice has greatly changed, including delivery processes, setting, organizational structure, and the roles and contributions of nurses and other health workers. Case management was introduced in the 1980s. Does case management improve health outcomes?

> Dominick Flarey, PhD, MBA, RN, CS, CNAA, FACHE: "Good systems of case management produce good outcomes...Time and time again, we see that containing costs generally results in poor outcomes, which brings patients back into the system in worse condition than when they first entered."

> Lucille Lombardi Travis, PhD, RN, CNA: "Data regarding the effects of the case management model are limited... Coordinated efforts are needed to identify the structures and processes of system implementation and evaluation so that outcome data can be brought together for systematic and collaborative outcomes analysis."

In Part II, the interviews of nursing leaders provide a contemporary context for understanding the changing landscape of nursing and health care, including critical social issues. They represent some of the many roles of nurses: the elected/appointed, the caregiver, the entrepreneur, the educator/administrator, and the historian. Their interviews highlight both their work in health care and in other arenas.

Imogene King and Diane O. McGivern are well known for their contributions to nursing theory and education, respectively. These interviews, however, focus on their contributions to the larger community outside of health care. King became politically active in the 1970s, when she tried to get a construction hole in her neighborhood—a danger to children, filled. She ended up being elected to the City Council herself. McGivern, in addition to heading the Division of Nursing at New York University, is Vice Chancellor of the New York Board of Regents—the governing body of the public school system in the state.

Eugene Sawicki is a doctorally prepared nurse and a priest. He brings his religious background to the healing process, adding a unique dimension to clinical practice. He uses this background to infuse the spiritual dimension into all that he does, to help patients "confront their dying, their immortality, and their need to make sense of where they are now."

Carolyn S. Zagury is founder, president, and owner of a publishing company. Her belief that nurses are talented, creative, and bold led her to take a risk to create a company to publish fiction and poetry by nurses. With no experience in the field, she says she "...did a lot of reading and talked to a friend. Then I just decided to go ahead and do it." She believes that her unique approach and entrepreneurial skills have made a difference.

Joan Lynaugh, a nurse historian, has influenced professional nursing through her work as an author, editor, professor, and the cofounder of the Center for the Study of History of Nursing. Her commitment to mentoring historians is fostered by the belief that "you can't have a movement with just one hand clapping. I mean you have to have people from every place 'get it.' If they don't 'get it,' you're not going to accomplish anything." How true this is of all the nurses whose ideas and beliefs are represented in *Nursing Leaders Speak Out*. Perhaps the future will be written differently based on the experiences and contributions of these leaders.

HARRIET R. FELDMAN
PHD, RN, FAAN

PART I

Point/Counterpoint on Contemporary Issues

Case Management: Is It Improving Health Outcomes?

Point: A System for Improving Outcomes

Dominick L. Flarey

Case management is a system that improves health outcomes. The jury is in on this one! Over the past decade we have witnessed and learned about the remarkable and stellar outcomes that are being realized through case management. Based on research and working with health care organizations nationally, I fully support the premise that case management works and that positive outcomes occur. While this statement is bold, it is also unique to certain systems and institutions. Of course, not all case management systems produce the same outcomes, and some systems have no effect on outcomes at all; however, good systems of case management produce good outcomes. Let's explore this further.

For positive outcomes to occur, case management systems must be designed appropriately. The first step in developing a quality case management system is to develop and support a vision of outcomes. My colleague, Dr. Suzanne Smith, and I have developed 10 major outcomes for any case management system. The outcomes to be achieved are: (1) cost effectiveness, (2) improvement in health status, (3) social responsiveness, (4) patient knowledge, (5) collaboration, (6) psychological equilibrium, (7) responsibility, (8) prevention, (9) provider knowledge, and (10) death with dignity (Flarey & Blancett, 1996).

Note: Originally published in *Nursing Leadership Forum*, Vol. 3, No. 4, 1998. New York: Springer Publishing Company.

To realize outcomes, you must first focus on them. In designing effective systems of case management, the key to success is defining the outcomes you want to achieve, and then planning backward to make them happen. In my experience, this is where most organizations fail. They simply start at the wrong place in systems development. They first develop some type of structure, decide who will "case manage" and then, at a later time, begin to assess outcomes. This approach is wrong and those who embrace it are doomed to failure. Case management can only work and produce positive outcomes when those outcomes have been predetermined. Anything short of this philosophy will likely produce poor results.

As such, it is safe to rephrase my previous statement and say that case management produces positive outcomes when the system has been designed correctly, i.e., with a focus on preplanned outcomes. There are other time-tested strategies that should be included in any systems design of case management. Case management systems that include such strategies and design elements, in my experience, are successful in achieving predetermined health outcomes. These include:

- Collaborative efforts in design and implementation
- Commitment to case management by the board of trustees and executive management
- Management of care delivery by professional registered nurses
- Physician education, participation, and support
- Multidisciplinary systems of case management
- Use of well-developed and tested pathways and protocol tools
- Intensive education for the entire health care team on the purpose of case management
- Patient/family involvement throughout the entire process of care delivery
- A system of variance tracking, trending, and analysis
- Comprehensive teaching programs for patients/families
- Expansion of case management across a continuum of care
- Integration of continuous quality improvement into the case management system.

The above are the keys to case management success. When these elements and strategies are in place, positive health outcomes result. The literature is clear in supporting these efforts and in documenting positive outcomes. Many case studies have been published that clearly demonstrate that outcomes are related to the quality of the case management systems design (Blancett & Flarey, 1998; Flarey & Blancett, 1998; Flarey & Blancett, 1996). Any organization developing case management would be wise to conduct a thorough review of the literature and abstract the key elements of systems that are producing stellar outcomes. Many organizations have been successful in providing a higher quality of care in cost-effective ways through case management systems. Their willingness to share their stories and strategies via published materials has been instrumental in our understanding of the "right" way to approach case management.

When critics claim that case management doesn't work, or does not produce positive health outcomes, I always question the system in place. I have seen and heard of case management systems that do not work. In analyzing such systems, a common thread is almost always noticeable. Poor systems of case management frequently do not have care being managed by qualified professional nurses, and most always emphasize cost containment and utilization management.

A large number of health care organizations have developed case management systems that look like this: A social worker provides for discharge planning and a registered nurse manages utilization of days, visits, etc. There is no focus or system in place to allow for the comprehensive management of patient care. Patients are usually seen as consumers "soaking up" health care dollars, and case management systems focus only on achieving cost and resource utilization reduction. These types of systems are doomed from the beginning.

The key to all predetermined outcomes for case management is the effectiveness of the system in managing comprehensive care. Time and time again, we see that containing costs generally results in poor outcomes, which brings patients back into the system in worse condition than when they first entered. Despite this frequent occurrence, many organizations continue in this manner and are at a loss to realize their mistakes.

In conclusion, I support the premise that good case management systems result in positive health outcomes. And poorly designed systems result in poor outcomes. It's a simple premise and one that is supported today in most of the literature on case management. Case management works when people develop it correctly, utilizing the strategies and key features discussed above. I firmly believe that case management is the delivery system of our time. "Case Management is the delivery system of the present and of the future. Yes, it too will change as all things do, but its basic concept, premises, and characteristics will stand the test of time for many years to come" (Flarey & Blancett, 1996, p. 14).

REFERENCES

Blancett, S. S., & Flarey, D. L. (1998). *Health care outcomes: Collaborative path-based approaches.* Gaithersburg, MD: Aspen Publishers Inc.

Flarey, D. L., & Blancett, S. S. (1996). *Handbook of nursing case management: Health care delivery in a world of managed care* (p. 14). Gaithersburg, MD: Aspen Publishers Inc.

Flarey, D. L., & Blancett, S. S. (1998). *Cardiovascular outcomes: Collaborative path-based approaches.* Gaithersburg, MD: Aspen Publishers Inc.

Counterpoint

Lucille Lombardi Travis

Well, maybe! The jury is still out. Case management gained prominence in the 1990s in response to modifications in the delivery of health care (Lynn & Kelley, 1998). Case management can be defined as a role, a technology, a process, a service, or all of these (Bower, 1992; Newell, 1996). Consequently, many models and definitions of case management have been adopted (Del Togno-Armanasco, Olivas, & Harter, 1989; Ethridge & Lamb, 1989; Lee, Mackenzie, Dudley-Brown, & Chin, 1998; May, Schraeder, & Britt, 1996; Zander, 1988). No matter what the definition or what the effectiveness measure, however, concern for outcomes has compelled health care professionals to intensify their efforts to produce evidenced-based practice. Data regarding the effects of the case management model, however, are limited.

As everyone knows, the health care industry is in a state of rapid and significant change. Historically, health care spending outpaced growth in the gross domestic product (GDP). Recently the rate of health care spending has slowed, so that its percentage of the GDP has stabilized (Williams & Torrens, 1999). Now, resounding concern for informed decision-making in health care by multiple constituents has directed the focus toward outcomes of care (Jones, Jennings, Moritz, & Moss, 1997). The value of the case management delivery method may be more easily recognizable if we change the wording from case management to outcomes management. This broadens the concept to encompass interdisciplinary aspects. It also reminds us that what we are interested in is outcomes—for the client first and foremost but also for the care delivery system (Wojner, 1996). Jones and associates (1997) identified five reasons to analyze outcomes:

> payers are demanding information about the results of care delivery; outcomes are an integral part of accreditation; consumers have a right to know about outcomes; regulatory agencies demand information about outcomes; and outcomes represent the basic reason for providing care. (p. 262)

In a time when system goals seem to outweigh client goals, case management can be seen as an avenue to identify individuals who might need a different approach to their care to obtain positive health outcomes (Bower, 1992). It has been stated, however, that conflict among the participants in case management, i.e., unequal power and opposing interests, can lead to problems for the individual charged with implementing case management (Padgett, 1998).

Some systems have incorporated strategies to overcome the problems often associated with case management. One health care institution that has developed a patient management system to improve selected outcomes through the use of advanced practice nurses is St. Luke's Episcopal Hospital in Houston, TX. Outcomes management is defined here as the utilization of outcomes assessment information to enhance clinical, quality, and financial outcomes. This approach utilizes quality and research vehicles to improve patient outcomes, thus balancing the cost-quality ratio. The person who implements the outcomes management is titled the "outcomes manager." The position has four subroles: clinical/consultation, research/quality, administrative/financial, and education. The ideal person to fill these roles is the advanced practice nurse, and at St. Luke's all outcomes managers are advanced practice nurses. The key to success of the position is an ability to document improvement of outcomes so that the institution values the patient management system. St. Luke's is an example of total organizational commitment to outcomes analysis, linking the results to tangible benefits (Houston & Luquire, 1997). This institution clearly embodies the implications for practice and management suggested by Jones and associates (1997).

In the broader framework of influencing policy, it is imperative that we as health care professionals continue to focus on outcomes evaluation. Studies of the effectiveness of case management as a care delivery system have typically focused on achievement of fiscal and clinical outcomes, and standardized nursing nomenclature is still being developed. I support the continued use of case management; however, coordinated efforts are needed to identify the structures and processes of system implementation and evaluation so that outcome data that have already been collected can be brought together for systematic and collaborative outcomes analysis. It is imperative that nursing continue to include, collect, and analyze data elements in patient databases. This attention to detail is facilitated by the use of information systems (Hale, 1995; Jones et al., 1997). Perhaps even more useful than case management as a care delivery method to improve patient outcomes is the use of information systems, which have contributed to our increased ability to organize, systematize, and track multiple aspects of care, enhancing the success of outcomes management.

In a continuously precarious health care arena, case management or, better said, outcomes management, may offer a window of opportunity to become a full partner in the effort to identify and implement evidence-based practice. This is where the potential of advanced practice nurses can be fully realized in coordinating care to produce positive outcomes.

REFERENCES

Bower, K. (1992). *Case management by nurses.* Washington, DC: American Nurses Publishing.

Del Togno-Armanasco, V., Olivas, G., & Harter, S. (1989). Developing an integrated nursing case management model. *Nursing Management, 20*(10), 26–29.

Ethridge, P., & Lamb, G. (1989). Professional nursing care management improves quality, access and costs. *Nursing Management, 20*(3), 30–35.

Hale, C. (1995). Research issues in case management. *Nursing Standard, 9*(44), 29–32.

Houston, S., & Luquire, R. (1997). Advanced practice nurse as outcomes manager. *Advanced Practice Nurse Quarterly, 3*(2), 1–9.

Jones, K., Jennings, B., Moritz, P., & Moss, M. (1997). Policy issues associated with analyzing outcomes of care. *Image: Journal of Nursing Scholarship, 29,* 261–267.

Lee, D., Mackenzie, A., Dudley-Brown, S., & Chin, T. (1998). Case management: A review of the definitions and practices. *Journal of Advanced Nursing, 27,* 933–939.

Lynn, M., & Kelley, B. (1998). Effects of case management on the nursing context-perceived quality of care, work satisfaction, and control over practice. *Image: Journal of Nursing Scholarship, 29,* 237–241.

May, C., Schraeder, C., & Britt, T. (1996). *Managed care & case management: Roles for professional nursing.* Washington, DC: American Nurses Publishing.

Newell, M. (1996). *Using nursing case management to improve health outcomes.* Frederick, MD: Aspen Publishers.

Padgett, S. (1998). Dilemmas of caring in a corporate context: A critique of nursing case management. *Advances in Nursing Science, 20*(4), 1–12.

Williams, S., & Torrens, P. (Eds.). (1999). *Introduction to health services.* Boston, MA: DelMar Publishers.

Wojner, A. (1996). Outcomes management: An interdisciplinary search for best practice. *AACN Clinical Issues: Advanced Practice in Acute and Critical Care, 7*(1), 133–145.

Zander, K. (1988). Nursing case management: Strategic management of cost and quality outcomes. *Journal of Nursing Administration, 18*(5), 23–30.

CHAPTER 2

Continuous Quality Improvement: Cult or Science?

Point: A New Philosophical Approach to Quality Assurance?

Janis P. Bellack

Over the last decade continuous quality improvement (CQI) has emerged to offer a broader framework for addressing quality of health care and health outcomes. From both a philosophical and practical perspective, CQI offers distinct advantages and improvements over the more familiar and widely used quality assurance (QA) approach to quality. CQI incorporates what is useful from QA but moves it to a new level, one that focuses on possibilities for improvement rather than simple oversight and compliance.

As a process, QA has not fulfilled its promise of assuring quality, largely because QA provides only for the assessment of quality, not its improvement. QA does not and cannot "assure" quality; it can only inspect it and make a judgment about it. Specifically, QA focuses on identifying problems in actual performance or outcomes, and whether certain standards have been adhered to. It assesses performance downstream, at a preestablished point in time, and makes a judgment about its effectiveness and efficiency—period! If quality is found deficient, QA offers no direction for what to do about it. Simply put, QA is not about assuring quality, only about inspecting it.

Note: Originally published in *Nursing Leadership Forum*, Vol. 4, No. 1, 1999. New York: Springer Publishing Company.

QA is beset by other limitations as well. Because it is externally initiated and driven, it tends to be a reactive rather than proactive process, a mechanism for responding to outside regulators and accreditors rather than to internal needs. Thus, QA is little more than an inspection and oversight process to assure compliance with external criteria and procedures. As such, it is often viewed as add-on work that must be done for someone else rather than a process with perceived benefits or one that is owned and valued by those in the organization or unit under review.

The QA approach often marginalizes accountability for quality because it is typically assigned to a designated QA department or a few compliance "watchdogs" instead of involving the entire organization. Such an arrangement also contributes to QA being viewed as an extra burden that bears little or no relation to daily work instead of being seen and valued as an important tool for improving daily work. Further, QA is frequently perceived as, and sometimes is, a way to find fault and fix blame if quality does not measure up to standards.

The very word *assurance* suggests that quality can be assured, which is misleading because quality itself cannot be guaranteed (Fanucci, Hammill, Johannson, Leggett, & Smith, 1993). Quality, however, can be assessed and improved. With its focus on continuous improvement, CQI offers a more encompassing, optimistic, and pragmatic approach to quality than does QA.

CQI evaluates performance and outcomes continuously along the way and not simply downstream. Most important, however, its findings are used as a basis for improving the upstream processes that produced deficiencies in performance or outcomes in the first place. Once the cause(s) of problems in performance or outcome are determined, small tests of change in upstream processes can be devised and tried in a series of Plan, Do, Study, and Act (PDSA) cycles to determine if they lead to improvements downstream, thus creating a cycle of continuous improvement (Guinane, Sikes, & Wilson, 1994; Langley, Nolan, & Nolan, 1994).

While both QA and CQI involve collecting and analyzing data, the former relies on data to decide if predetermined standards have been met, whereas the latter uses data as a basis for making improvements (change) in a system. QA's focus on collecting endpoint data to determine only whether threshold standards have been met limits its potential usefulness. While QA may be an effective measure of current conditions (what is), it does not provide a broader framework for using what was learned from the data to change the system or its processes in order to improve performance or outcomes (what can be).

CQI operates within a framework of system thinking that takes into account the interactions and interrelationships among all components of a system. With its focus on systems instead of individuals, CQI fosters an organizational culture in which problems are treated as system errors rather than individual errors, and thus, as opportunities for improvement. A CQI approach to quality recognizes that problems in a system are often beyond the ability of an individual to fix because the problems are inherent in the system and not the fault of individuals. Most significantly, CQI goes beyond identifying problems and uses the data and findings to guide actions toward improvement. Thus, problems are seen as *opportunities* to work together for improvement rather than finding individual fault, resulting in a more positive organizational climate and better morale.

As an approach to quality, CQI also acknowledges the contributions to quality made by all members of the organization. The processes, language, and tools of CQI are not the province of one discipline or department but can be shared by all. Responsibility and accountability are also shared. Successful CQI depends on involving as many people as possible and not delegating responsibility for quality to a few designated quality officers or a QA department.

FIGURE 2.1 Contrasting CQI and QA.

Continuous Quality Improvement	Quality Assurance
Internally driven	Externally dictated
Prospective	Retrospective
Proactive	Reactive
System focused	Individual focused
Improvement (what can be)	Inspection (what is)
Drives out fear (à la Deming[1])	Places blame (à la Dilbert[2])
Continuous	Periodic
Interdisciplinary	Separate disciplines
Part of daily operations	Separate from daily operations

[1] Deming, W. E. (1986). *Out of the Crisis*. Boston: Massachusetts Institute of Technology Press.
[2] Adams, S. (1994). *The Dilbert Principle*. New York: Harper.

A shift to CQI does not mean that the need for periodic inspection and evaluation by external regulators and accreditors will go away. It does mean, however, that the organization—and those who work in it—take responsibility for producing quality performance and outcomes in their daily operations and hold themselves accountable for doing so. A fully developed and integrated system of CQI may even make it possible one day to eliminate the laborious, time-consuming, and expensive process of preparing for external accreditation. Instead, external accreditors and regulators adopt a CQI approach to assessing organizational quality. This would transform the current focus on inspection and compliance to determining whether the organization has an effective internal system in place for evaluating and continuously improving its processes, performance, and outcomes. With such a system, processes are always in place and always operating to continuously improve quality; thus, the system is prepared for review at any time.

In conclusion, a CQI approach to quality offers numerous advantages over QA (see Figure 2.1). Clearly, CQI delivers a comprehensive, optimistic, future-oriented, integrated, and sustainable approach for evaluating quality and taking action to assure—not quality itself—but its continuous improvement.

REFERENCES

Fanucci, D., Hammill, M., Johannson, P., Leggett, J., & Smith, M. J. (1993). Quantum leap into continuous quality improvement. *Nursing Management, 24*(6), 28–30.

Guinane, C. S., Sikes, J. I., & Wilson, R. K. (1994). Using the PDSA cycle to standardize a quality assurance program in a quality improvement-driven environment. *The Joint Commission Journal on Quality Improvement, 20*, 696–705.

Langley, G. J., Nolan, K. M., & Nolan, T. W. (1994, June). The foundation of improvement. *Quality Progress, 27*, 81–86.

Counterpoint

Farrokh Alemi

Continuous Quality Improvement (CQI) has received widespread acceptance in health care. Use of CQI raises an obvious question: Does it work? Or more specifically, does the CQI effort improve an organization's productivity and viability? Many studies show the success of different CQI projects (Bluth, Havrilla, & Blakeman, 1993; Kibbe, Bentz, & McLaughlin, 1993; McEachern, Makens, Buchanan, & Schiff, 1991; McGarvey & Harper, 1993; Pachciarz, Abbot, Gorman, Henneman, & Kuhl, 1992; Parenti, Lederle, Impola, & Peterson, 1994; Schafer, 1994; Young, Ward, & McCarthy, 1994). Others (U.S. General Accounting Office, 1991) point to organizations that have improved their revenue or productivity after implementing CQI. These studies do not constitute ample evidence of CQI effectiveness and projects that fail are not reported. Focusing on success and ignoring failures creates an unbalanced view of the potential for CQI to bring about change.

A few investigators have tried to evaluate the effectiveness of CQI across organizations. In a survey of non-healthcare organizations, managers believed that most CQI efforts have not been effective and that two thirds of CQI efforts have ground to a halt (Senge, 1990). A Gallop survey of American executives (1989) shows that only 28% believe that their CQI efforts have led to changes in market share or have increased profitability. In the health care arena, when CEOs and directors of quality assurance/improvement departments in 61 hospitals were asked about the impact of their CQI efforts, they perceived that these efforts led to better patient outcomes but not to better financial outcomes. One study also examined objective measures of clinical efficiency (severity-adjusted length of stay and charges) in 38 hospitals and found no relationship between the measures and CQI implementation, when adjusting for other hospital characteristics such as size of the hospital (Shortell et al., 1995).

Studies in which randomized assignment has been used, i.e., studies that are most likely to have valid findings about the effectiveness of CQI, with some exceptions (Curley, McEachern, & Speroff, 1998) have reached similar conclusions. In a randomized, controlled trial of 15 clinics (95 providers, 4995 patients), implementation of CQI for management of hypertensive patients had no impact on patient outcomes (Goldberg et al., 1998). A recent review of randomized studies concluded: "The few randomized studies suggest no impact of CQI on clinical outcomes and no evidence to date of organization-wide improvement in clinical performance" (Shortell, Bennett, & Byck, 1998). Naturally, organizations differ to the extent that they have implemented the CQI process. CQI has become an amorphous method that seems to include diverse approaches ranging from a philosophy to a specific mathematical technique (Gann & Restuccia, 1994).

One wonders: How did we get here? Why have so many people adopted a process that is uncertain to work? Given a lack of data on the effectiveness of CQI, and lack of an accepted definition of CQI, it is suprising that so many have adopted the CQI process. "It is amusing that a technique that argues for making decisions based on evidence depends so strongly on elements of faith" (personal communication with Giorgio Piccagli, 1994). Common sense suggests that CQI: (1) blames the system, not the people; (2) studies the process, acts and reexamines; (3) involves all employees in improvement; (4) relies on information and benchmarking; and (5) uses cross-functional teams. But are these ideas supported with research? A recent study found support for some of these principles (Gustafson & Hundt, 1995); however, it seems that these principles are accepted because they are reasonable, not because they are based on research.

On the surface it is hard to even conjecture arguments against these principles. They seem so obvious, which may be why CQI has been implemented throughout many organizations without asking whether the approach really works. The real test for ideas and their appropriateness is an empirical one. Neither the popularity nor the simplicity of the idea tells us much about its validity. What we need is empirical evidence that organizations are able to implement the proposed ideas and that implementation (with all its diversity) leads to positive change, predominantly measured in terms of organization growth and productivity. Without such evidence, management will swing from one set of common-sense ideas to another, always worrying about what organizational change method will be the next fashion.

Can the principles of CQI be defended based on extant empirical data? At the present time, the answer is no. Some of the attributes of CQI are discussed below. I argue that despite their merits they are not always appropriate.

- Blame the system, not the people. The logic of this principle is simple, i.e., take away fear and you create a trusting environment for employees to experiment with change.

    Data show that layoffs, i.e., blaming people and not the system, can sometimes lead to both improved motivation on the part of remaining employees and improved productivity (Brockner, Grover, Reed, & Dewitt, 1992; Kraft, 1991). CQI fails to address adequately the possibility of changing organizations through changing personnel. By assuming that employees are to retain their current positions, CQI ignores the possibility of substituting physicians with less expensive professionals or technology, a well-documented source of savings. Thus, it ignores a central method of improving productivity.

    CQI assumes that when employees' skills do not fit the proposed change, the employees should be retrained. This may make sense in manufacturing but not in health care. In health care, where employees already have extensive and specialized education, retraining may be a poor fit. For example, if we have decided to rely more heavily on nurse practitioners, it would be unreasonable to train a physician to become a nurse. Deming's (1984) concept of retraining employees makes sense if we are talking about unskilled laborers who can be retrained in a limited time. In health care, where many employees are extensively trained and are committed to their careers, retraining seems pointless.

- Study the process, act, and reexamine. CQI encourages participants to draw detailed flow charts of activities before searching for solutions. For example, to reduce Cesarean birth rates, examine what happens to the patient as she enters the hospital until the Cesarean is done, then suggest solutions. Flow charts are drawn showing the flow of work. Fish bone diagrams are made of the causes of Cesarean section.

    Does it make sense to understand a process in so much detail before searching for solutions? No. Research on planning suggests generating solutions before understanding the constraints of the process in detail. In this way, one's imagination shifts from "what is" to "what could be." Once a solution is selected, it is reviewed to see how the solution should be adjusted to fit the constraint of the workflow. Nadler (1970) calls this process of problem solving the "Ideal System design." The Ideal System design and CQI processes aim to determine practical solutions. Both fit the solutions to the features of the underlying process, but in the Ideal System design this is done at the end while in the CQI it is done at the beginning.

Does it really matter, when we examine the real life constraints? Yes, it does. In research conducted on planning, data show that brainstorming about the ideal solutions and fitting them to reality at a later stage lead to more effective ideas (Nutt, 1977). CQI encourages anchoring to what exists, rather than to what can be. The latter is a more creative starting point.

- Total employee involvement. A rationale for increased participation of employees is that participation will lead to increased employee satisfaction and, consequently, higher productivity. There is substantial support for the effect of participation on the successful implementation of change. Employees are more likely to implement ideas that they work on and invest in. In addition, employee participation improves morale and satisfaction (Conte, Glandon, Oleske, & Hill, 1992).

  Data from research on organizational development and changing employees' experience of work suggest another relationship. Increases in productivity may be associated with lower satisfaction with work (Zyzanski, Stange, Langa, & Flocke, 1998).

- Cross-functional teams. Advocates of CQI argue that cross-functional teams of employees should be involved in proposing change in order to make sure that the team understands the whole system. Presumably involving cross-functional teams helps improve the quality of the solution and reduce implementation difficulties.

  In a recent study of 131 hospitals (Pinto, Pinto, & Prescott, 1993), cooperation among cross-functional teams led to more satisfaction with the group process but did not lead to success as measured by the team members themselves. Contrary to expected CQI outcomes, cooperation among cross-functional teams was not related to more successful projects.

Another problem with cross-functional teams of employees is that, no matter what the function, employees have a stake in the status quo. At different stages in problem-solving it is a good idea to involve different types of people (Nutt, 1976), some from outside the organization. CQI uses internal teams to plan change. When both employees and outside experts are involved at different points in the team's deliberations, the quality of the solution and the likelihood of success improve.

CONCLUSION

This counterpoint position is intended to convey that some very basic and familiar principles of CQI cannot be defended based solely on anecdotal evidence from the field. This is not to say that CQI is not effective, nor that we should abandon efforts to employ this strategy. Instead, we need to look closely at the evidence on CQI as well as other models of change. The spread of CQI has been remarkable. It has focused our attention on service delivery improvements and allowed management to participate in clinical decisions. I believe it is now time to focus our attention on how CQI or any other organizational process can produce successful organization-wide results. Without such inspection, quality improvement will become a "cult" or passing trend, rather than a practice based on rational science.

REFERENCES

American Society for Quality Control. (1989). *Quality: Executive priority or afterthought?* A survey conducted by the Gallop organization for the American Society for Quality Control. Milwaukee, WI: Author.

Bluth, E. I., Havrilla, M., & Blakeman, C. (1993). Quality improvement techniques: Value to improve the timeliness of preoperative chest radiographic reports. *American Journal of Radiology, 160,* 995–998.

Brockner, J., Grover, S., Reed, T. F., & Dewitt, R. S. (1992). Layoffs, job insecurity, and survivors work effort: Evidence of an inverted U relationship. *Academy of Management, 35*, 413–425.

Conte, M. A., Glandon, G. L., Oleske, D. M., & Hill, J. P. (1992). Total quality management in a health care organization: How are employees affected? *Hospital & Health Services Administration, 37*, 503–518.

Curley, C., McEachern, J. E., & Speroff, T. (1998, August). A firm trial of interdisciplinary rounds on the inpatient medical wards: An intervention designed using continuous quality improvement. *Medical Care, 36*(Suppl. 8), AS4–AS12.

Deming, W. E. (1984). *Quality, productivity and competitive position.* Cambridge, MA: Massachusetts Institute of Technology.

Gann, M. J., & Restuccia, J. D. (1994). Total quality management: A view of current and potential research. *Medical Care Review, 51*, 467–500.

Goldberg, H. I., Wagner, E. H., Fihn, S. D., Martin, D. P., Horowitz, C. R., Christensen, D. B., Cheadle, A. D., Diehr, P., & Simon, G. (1998). A randomized controlled trial of CQI teams and academic detailing: Can they alter compliance with guidelines? *Joint Commission Journal of Quality Improvement, 24*(3), 130–142.

Gustafson, D. H., & Hundt, A. S. (1995, Spring). Findings of innovation research applied to quality management principles for health care. *Health Care Management Review, 20*(2), 16–33.

Kibbe, D. C., Bentz, E., & McLaughlin, C. P. (1993). Continuous quality improvement for continuity of care. *Journal of Family Practice, 36*, 304–308.

Kraft, K. (1991). The incentive effects of dismissals, efficiency wages, piece-rate and profit sharing. *Review of Economics and Statistics, 73*, 451–459.

McEachern, J. E., Makens, P. K., Buchanan, E. D., & Schiff, L. (1991). Quality improvement: An imperative for medical care. *Journal of Occupational Medicine, 33*, 364–373.

McGarvey, R. N., & Harper, J. J. (1993). Pneumonia mortality reduction and quality improvement in a community hospital. *Quality Review Bulletin, 19*, 124–130.

Nadler, G. (1970). *Work system design.* New York: Irwin.

Nutt, P. C. (1977). An experimental comparison of the effectiveness of three planning methods. *Management Science, 23*, 499–511.

Nutt, P. C. (1976). The merits of using consumers and experts as members of planning groups. *Academy of Management Journal, 19,* 378–394.

Pachciarz, J. A., Abbot, M. I., Gorman, B., Henneman, C. E., & Kuhl, M. (1992). Continuous quality improvement of Pap smears in an ambulatory care facility. *Quality Review Bulletin, 18,* 229–235.

Parenti, C. M., Lederle, F. A., Impola, C. L., & Peterson, L. R. (1994). Reduction of unnecessary intravenous catheter use: Internal medicine house staff participate in a successful quality improvement project. *Archives of Internal Medicine, 154,* 1829–1832.

Pinto, M. B., Pinto, J. K., & Prescott, J. E. (1993). Antecedents and consequences of project team cross-functional consequences. *Management Science, 39,* 1281–1296.

Shafer, D. (1994) Healthier babies in Twin Falls, Idaho: A case study. *Journal of Health Administration Education, 12,* 319–330.

Senge, P. M. (1990). *The fifth discipline: The art and practice of the learning organization.* New York: Currency Doubleday.

Shortell, S. M., Bennett, C. L., & Byck, G. R. (1998). Assessing the impact of continuous quality improvement on clinical practice: What it will take to accelerate progress. *Milbank Quarterly, 76,* 593–624.

Shortell, S. M., O'Brien, J. L., Carman, J. M., Foster, R. W., Hughes, E. F. X., Boerstler, H., & O'Conner, E. J. (1995). Assessing the impact of continuous quality improvement/total quality management: Concept versus implementation. *Health Services Research, 30,* 377–401.

U.S. General Accounting Office. (1991, May). *Management practices: U.S. companies improve performance through quality efforts* (GAO/NSIAD-91-190). Washington, DC: Author.

Young, M. J., Ward, R., & McCarthy, B. (1994). Continuously improving primary care. *Joint Commission Journal on Quality Improvement, 20,* 120–126.

Zyzanski, S. J., Stange, K. C., Langa, D., & Flocke, S. A. (1998, May). Trade-offs in high-volume primary care practice. *Journal of Family Practice, 46,* 397–402.

education or conceptual framework. It means that ". . . we need to understand how others see the world, their motivations, emotions, and aspirations. To see a problem in a new light, we need to analyze it from perspectives other than our own . . . to put ourselves in other people's shoes and to see the world from their point of view" (Fisher, Kopelman, & Schneider, 1994, p. 21). While this has obvious implications for the current flurry of redesign activities, it has broader implications for survival in a time of fiscal constraint.

EDUCATIONAL PERSPECTIVES

Those returning to school to obtain advanced academic credentials need to understand that, while their reasons for wanting an advanced education might be the same as they've always been for nurses, the expectations and eventual outcomes will be radically different. In the past, some nurses may have returned for a graduate degree simply because their employer provided tuition reimbursement benefits. This was also a time when such benefits were provided on a tax-free basis. Current budget constraints and changes in tax laws have resulted in greatly reduced or restricted tuition reimbursement benefits. Some institutions will now reimburse only for those programs that directly relate to the employee's role. This means that potential students need to have a clear idea of their role preparation and its expected outcome *before* they begin. In this way, students can choose programs wisely, and can communicate their needs so that faculty can more specifically structure the educational experience, especially clinical practice.

Regardless of specialty, preparation for a graduate degree should include the development of critical thinking skills, data management skills, and platform skills that allow the graduate to act as an organizational citizen in a new, highly competitive environment. With these skills, the graduate will not only be able to enact role implementation at a high level, but will also be equipped to communicate needs, activities, and information in a way that enables a meaningful response. Articulation of these needs may relate to those of the graduate's constituency or may be related to the nurse's own needs for development.

CHAPTER *3*

Genetics Counseling: Should It Be a Basic Competency for Nurses?

Point

Constance Visovsky

In light of the explosive advances made in genetics recently, it would not be difficult to imagine the following scenario. A 43-year-old woman who underwent genetic testing has been diagnosed with familial hypercholesterolemia. She presents to the clinic for a follow-up visit accompanied by her overweight 13-year-old son. She has made a list of questions for the nurse regarding the implications of the genetic information she has received. Can the nurse in the clinic help this client? Are nurses prepared for the inevitable shift in practice that genetic biotechnology will bring? If not, they should be.

In 1990, the international research program known as the Human Genome Project was established. The goal of the project is to analyze the structure of human DNA (deoxyribonucleic acid) and determine the location and sequence of 50,000–100,000 human genes (Department of Health and Human Services, Public Health Service National Institutes of Health, 1995). The advent of the Human Genome Project has heralded changes in health care delivery as our knowledge of the disease process expands. As new knowledge is generated about the genetic basis of common disease states, genetic

Note: Originally published in *Nursing Leadership Forum*, Vol. 4, No. 2, 1998. New York: Springer Publishing Company.

testing for disease is becoming increasingly prevalent. New treatment options in the form of gene therapy portend to become more common in the clinical setting. Nurses must now be prepared to meet the challenges of incorporating an understanding of this new technology into their everyday practice.

Genetic counseling has been defined as "a communication process which deals with the human problems associated with the occurrence, or risk of occurrence, of a genetic disorder in a family" (Scott, 1998, p. 285). The purpose of genetic counseling is to assist the individual and family to: (1) understand the disorder and management options, (2) understand the role of heredity in the disorder, (3) understand the implications for managing the risk of occurrence, and (4) assist in adjustment to the disorder, or to the risk of recurrence of the disorder (Scott, 1998). Practicing nurses provide counseling services to their clients. Nurses routinely perform risk assessments, educate clients and families concerning disease states and treatment plans, and assist them in coping with the psychological consequences of disease. Expanding this role to include genetic counseling appears to be a reasonable evolution. Nurses enjoy access to clients in a variety of settings. Thus, clinical nurses are ideally poised to assume an important role in genetic counseling.

Advances in genetic biotechnology have clinical, ethical, and professional implications for nurses. In 1995, the American Nurses Association (ANA) reaffirmed its position that nursing is a scientific discipline that uses both basic and applied knowledge (ANA, 1995). In order to maintain acceptable standards of practice in the clinical arena, nurses must keep pace with advancing health care technologies and their implications for health care delivery (Monsen & Anderson, 1999). New discoveries in genetic technology will require nurses to begin incorporating these advances in health care technology into the practice arena. Nurses will be called upon to provide preventive education, referrals, and counseling services to clients (Foley & Sommers, 1998).

According to Monsen and Anderson (1999), every nurse should be prepared with basic competencies in genetics in order to perform health assessments, identify at-risk individuals, provide case management and educational services, and assist clients with genetic testing decision-making. In addition, nurses will require an understanding of genetics to prevent unauthorized use of confidential genetic information. Nurses will play an important role in educating the public regarding the delicate nature of genetic information and the necessary privacy protections (Scanlon & Fibson, 1995). Armed with genetic counseling competencies, nurses can determine outcomes for clients achievable by nursing interventions. Knowledge deficit, anxiety control, and risk detection are examples of interventions that can be implemented by nurses (Johnson & Maas, 1997).

The actions of health professionals are guided by certain ethical principles. Nurses have an ethical obligation to be educated in genetic biotechnology, as advances in this area can impact client care, public health, and participation in genetic research. As nurses are well positioned to participate in genetic counseling, they have a moral obligation to educate clients and their families. The principle of autonomy demands that nurses inform their clients about issues associated with genetic testing, such as potential risks and benefits, confidentiality, and health insurance implications (Dwyer, 1998). Nurses can assess a client's understanding of information, assist with clarification of values and goals, and offer support for their decisions (Scanlon & Fibson, 1995). The principle of justice confers the right to fair and equitable treatment. Nurses in case management positions can invoke the principle of justice by acting to ensure equal access and distribution of genetic services.

Last, as indicated by the principle of nonmaleficence, health care professionals should "do no harm." The underlying premise here is that the health care professional should therefore "do good." Nurses have the potential to positively impact the care of those individuals seeking genetic services. Nurses understand the issues of disease impact, quality of life, the cost-benefit ratio of genetic biotechnology, and the health insurance implications associated with it. Nursing interventions in a trusting client-nurse relationship can promote a person's good through genetic counseling, education, and support services (Dwyer, 1998).

The professional implications of genetic biotechnology in the health care system abound. The role of the professional nurse providing care in an era of rampant genetic advances has not yet been defined (Jenkins, 1997). Genetics is an area ripe for the development of health policy that requires a nursing perspective. There are issues surrounding access to genetic information and testing, protection of client confidentiality, informed consent and decision-making, as well as allocation of funds for genetically based research programs.

In order for the nursing profession to influence health policy in any meaningful way, educational preparation for nurses must include genetics courses at both the basic and advanced levels (Jenkins, 1997). Nurses in particular need adequate understanding of molecular genetics to assist their clients with the overwhelming amount of genetic information available. To meet this goal, schools of nursing must respond by integrating genetics into their curricula, thus preparing nurses to integrate genetic principles into their care of clients. Health care organizations too must respond by incorporating basic genetic counseling competencies into their continuing education programs for nurses. It is through education that nurses can be adequately prepared to impact genetic health policies.

In the past, individuals with genetic disorders were in the care of genetic specialists. Today, health care professionals will encounter clients with genetic disorders in all practice settings. As scientists continue in their endeavor to map the human genome, nurses at the bedside can and should expand their role to include genetic counseling. It is incumbent upon nurses to take the lead in defining their role in this biotechnical age. The time is ripe for nurses to expand their skills, develop new roles, and influence the manner in which genetic services are delivered now and in the future.

REFERENCES

American Nurses Association. (1995). *Social policy statement.* Washington, DC: Author.

Department of Health and Human Services, Public Health Services, National Institutes of Health. (1995). *The Human Genome Project: From maps to medicine* (NIH Publication No. 96-3897). Bethesda, MD: National Center for Human Genome Research.

Dwyer, M. (1998). Genetic research and ethical challenges: Implications for nursing practice. *AACN Clinical Issues, 9*(4), 600–605.

Foley, S., & Sommers, M. (1998). Molecular genetics: From bench to bedside. *AACN Clinical Issues, 9*(4), 491–498.

Jenkins, J. (1997). Educational issues related to cancer genetics. *Seminars in Oncology Nursing, 13*(2), 141–144.

Johnson, M., & Maas, M. (1997). *Iowa outcomes project: Nursing outcomes project (NOC).* St. Louis: Mosby.

Monsen, R., & Anderson, G. (1999). Continuing education for nurses that incorporates genetics. *The Journal of Continuing Education in Nursing, 30*(1), 20–24.

Scanlon, C., & Fibson, W. (1995). *Managing genetic information: Implications for nursing practice.* Washington, DC: American Nurses Association.

Scott, J. A. (1998). Genetic counseling. In J. A. Scott (Ed.), *Genetic applications: A health perspective* (pp. 285–291). Lawrence, KS: Learner Managed Designs.

Counterpoint: Good Intentions Do Not Absolve Misinformation

M. Linda Workman

One of the hottest topics in nursing and medicine today is the role of genetics in susceptibility to specific diseases. Many common health problems are not equal opportunity employers and have a genetic basis for increased risk of development. Such health problems include coronary artery disease, diabetes mellitus, breast cancer, and rheumatoid arthritis, to name only a few. The fact that these disorders have only recently been acknowledged to have a genetic predisposition demonstrates the confounding issue of genetic influence not always following the strict Mendelian rules for patterns of inheritance currently associated with such disorders as Huntington's disease, Sickle Cell disease, or classic hemophilia. Rather, genetic predisposition represents one part of the equation requisite for disease development. The multifactorial interactions among genetic predisposition, environmental influences, and lifestyle choices together determine whether the inherited risk is ever expressed during a person's lifetime and to what degree (disease severity) (Gregersen, 1997). Thus, analysis of whether or not a specific gene has been inherited cannot alone determine individual risk, making genetic counseling of "at-risk" individuals a complicated and daunting task requiring specialized knowledge well beyond the scope of basic nursing education (Dimond, Calzone, Davis, & Jenkins, 1998; International Society of Nurses in Genetics, Inc., 1998).

The current definition of genetic counseling, based on a human genetics model rather than a behavioral science model and adopted by the American Society of Human Genetics, is the gold standard by which genetic counselors are expected to practice and by which criteria for reimbursement are set. This definition is:

> Genetic counseling is a communication process which deals with the human problems associated with the occurrence or risk of occurrence of a genetic disorder within a family. This process

involves an attempt by one or more appropriately trained persons to help the individual or family to:

1. comprehend the medical facts including the medical diagnosis, probable course of the disorder, and the available management;
2. appreciate the way heredity contributes to the disorder and the risk of recurrence in specified relatives;
3. understand the alternatives for dealing with the risk of recurrence;
4. choose a course of action which seems to them appropriate in their view of their risk, their family goals, and their ethical and religious standards and act in accordance with that decision; and
5. make the best possible adjustment to the disorder in an affected family member and/or to the risk of recurrence of that disorder. (Jorde, Carey, Bamshad, & White, 1999, p. 292)

This definition, while encompassing some of the formal and informal roles assumed by registered nurses, stipulates that the professional performing genetic counseling has documented expertise and evidence of advanced education in this specialty. Neither the basic educational program for nursing nor that of medicine fulfills the degree of specialization needed for genetics counseling (Kenner, 1998).

The calculation of odds ratios for personal risk of any disorder that carries some degree of genetic predisposition requires in-depth understanding of population genetics, Bayesian analysis, molecular genetics, Mendelian patterns of inheritance, and epigenetic events regulating gene expression. Counseling of any type requires grounding in behavioral sciences, psycho-social issues, and communication skills. Certified genetic counselors must first earn a master's degree in a recognized genetic counseling program that includes focused specialty content delivered in classroom, clinical, and laboratory settings and then pass a national certifying examination.

Nurses have long been patient advocates as well as interpreters of medical language and purpose. It is of nurses that patients feel most free to ask questions and from whom they expect honest, understandable answers. It is also the nurse who spends the most time listening and piecing together family history and other pertinent background information. Nurses are viewed as formal and informal counselors in assisting patients to be informed consumers of health care. Therefore, a natural extension of this role would seem to be that of genetic counseling. The problem with such an extension, however, is the dearth of preparation and information most nurses have regarding the science of genetics and intricacies of genetic expression.

During the past decade, increasing numbers of specialty and advanced practice nurses have recognized the role of genetics in the pathogenesis of many diseases. These same nurses have also recognized the level of detail regarding genetics missing from both basic nursing education and most advanced nursing education programs. Continuing education programs and focused self-study have assisted specialty and advanced practice nurses to acquire a beginning level knowledge base from which to identify individuals at genetic risk; however, relatively few nurses, even advanced practice nurses, have become sufficiently grounded to practice genetic counseling. This dearth is related to exposure and education rather than to ability.

Historically, nurses have been expected to assume many duties for which they have been minimally prepared during their basic education. For example, nurses are expected to be as familiar with the medications they administer as the physician who prescribes them and the pharmacist who dispenses them. Moreover, nurses are expected to identify prescribing and dispensing errors made by other health professionals. Many nursing programs, however, do not have a formal pharmacology course or only require a single 2-credit course to cover this content at a relatively superficial level. Teaching patients and families about dietary modifications needed for people with different types of metabolic problems is another example of nurses applying specialty principles that were presented at a minimal level in basic nursing education.

As the demands of nursing practice increase and greater genetic involvement is identified in disease pathogenesis, more pressure is placed on the nurse to take an active role in one or more aspects of genetic counseling. In spite of enormous advances in the understanding of genetic mechanisms, genetics content in basic nursing education has not kept pace with medical science and has scarcely changed in 30 years. The typical basic nursing program presents genetic content for a total of 3 to 12 clock-hours as part of a biological science course. The trend is changing at advanced practice and specialty levels toward increasing genetics preparation for those nurses working at the forefront of this specialty (International Society of Nurses in Genetics, Inc., 1998; Kelly, 1993; Sommers, Hetteberg, Kenner, & Prows, 1998). Nurses are increasing their involvement in genetics at the national level by establishing organizations that target genetics and nursing, such as the International Society of Nurses in Genetics (ISONG), the Genetics Special Interest Group of the Oncology Nursing Society, and organizations that are attempting to change genetics content in health professional education, such as the National Coalition for Health Professional Education in Genetics (NCHPEG) (Kenner, 1998). The National Institute for Nursing Research has made greater involvement of nursing with issues related to genetics a priority for the next millennium (Sigmon, Grady, & Amende, 1997).

The issue is not whether nurses *can* perform genetic counseling but rather *should* they perform genetic counseling, given the minimal genetics preparation available in most basic nursing programs. Failing to accurately identify people at risk or to miscalculate odds ratios that result in the engendering of unnecessary anxiety and fear is not helpful, regardless of the intention to provide the best care. Giving nurses the responsibility of genetic counseling without providing them with the tools of authority (adequate education) is a recipe for disaster and opens the discipline to criticism. Major changes in nursing education are essential before genetic counseling has the potential to be a basic nursing competency.

REFERENCES

Dimond, E., Calzone, K., Davis, J., & Jenkins, J. (1998). Programmed instruction: The role of the nurse in cancer genetics. *Cancer Nursing, 21*(1), 57–70.

Gregersen, P. (1997). Genetic analysis of rheumatic disease. In W. Kelley, E. Harris, S. Ruddy, & C. Sledge (Eds.), *Textbook of rheumatology* (5th ed., pp. 209–216). Philadelphia: W. B. Saunders.

International Society of Nurses in Genetics, Inc. (1998). *Statement on the scope and standards of genetics clinical nursing practice.* Washington, DC: American Nurses Publishing.

Jorde, L. B., Carey, J. C., Bamshad, M. J., & White, R. L. (1999). *Medical genetics* (2nd ed.). St. Louis: C. V. Mosby.

Kelly, P. (1993). Breast cancer risk: The role of the nurse practitioner. *Nurse Practitioner Forum, 4*(2), 91–95.

Kenner, C. (1998). National coalition for health professional education in genetics. *AACN Clinical Issues: Advanced Practice in Acute and Critical Care, 9*(4), 582–587.

Sigmon, H., Grady, P. A., & Amende, L. M. (1997). The National Institute of Nursing Research explores opportunities in genetics research. *Nursing Outlook, 45*, 215–219.

Sommers, M. S., Hetteberg, C., Kenner, C., & Prows, C. (1998). Genetics and Nursing: Searching for a role in a revolution. *AACN Clinical Issues: Advanced Practice in Acute and Critical Care, 9*(4), 465–466.

CHAPTER 4

The Shift of Acute Care From the Hospital to the Home: Is It a Good Trend?

Point

Christine A. Pierce

Home health care, as an alternative to hospital care, has received unprecedented media attention over the last few years. Unfortunately, most of it has not been positive. Spurred by reports of overutilization and fraud, and purported to justify the disproportionate reimbursement cuts associated with the Balanced Budget Act of 1997 (BBA '97), this negative perspective of the home health industry has overshadowed the many positive outcomes of patient care within this specialty.

Although the provision of community-based care has a long history in the public health and visiting nurse movements, home health care as an alternative to acute institutional care is a relatively recent refocus of the 1965 Medicare home health benefit. The original intent was to expand services through which patients could receive mid- to longer-term care beyond the more critical stages. Today's trend is toward the placement of early discharge, acute cases—so-called "quicker and sicker"—into home care as an alternative to hospital care.

From 1993 to 1996 the number of hospital-based home health care agencies grew exponentially. This is attributable to a number of factors, including: (1) constrained reimbursement for in-patient

Note: Originally published in *Nursing Leadership Forum*, Vol. 4, No. 3, 2000. New York: Springer Publishing Company.

care resulting in tighter utilization management and a decreasing length of hospital stay (LOS); (2) a trend among health systems to cast a wider net of control over patients within their catchment areas, securing them to the health system for all needs, thus requiring that the continuity of health care management expand beyond institutional walls; (3) increased consumer awareness, therefore demand of health care services within the comfort and familiarity of home, and (4) provider reimbursement advantages, especially within the cost-based framework of Medicare, for the delivery of home health services. A growing elderly population has assured the steady availability of patients with complex health care needs that exceed an average 5-day hospital stay, giving rise to questions concerning the effectiveness and value of home health care as an alternative to the hospital.

Although aspects of hospital care will most likely always be essential, the shift of patients to home health care is beneficial from a number of perspectives—not the least of which is avoidance of the inherent risks of an in-patient stay. From the first class on fundamentals of patient care, nursing professionals have been wary of the potential institutional hazards of nosocomial infection and iatrogenically induced complications. Separating a patient from the familiar surroundings of the home environment and social support systems has a depersonalizing effect that can result in dependence, mental status changes, and less than active participation in one's recovery. The focus of ever-shortening hospital stays is understandably the current illness or condition, but due to scarce time and few resources, there is a risk of neglecting to holistically place the event within the overall context of that patient's health and wellness.

Enter the home setting: the patient's familiar domain, free of institutional "bugs," an information-packed environment from which the care plan can be jointly crafted to address the patient's real life from the perspective of those who live it. It is here that the magic of nurse/patient/caregiver partnering can truly materialize, and where the investigative processes of nursing science can yield an abundance of important information that might otherwise go undetected, thus not addressed. Seeing the patients' world from their viewpoints facilitates the development of realistic goals and fosters their participation in achieving positive outcomes. It facilitates patient and caregiver learning within an environment that is generally less stressful than that of the hospital, thus hastening independence. Successful care at home builds patients' confidence in the ongoing management of their health and illness by reinforcing self-care abilities.

Acute problems that previously required significant hospital stays, such as febrile neutropenia (Talcott, Whalen, Clark, Rieker, & Finberg, 1994) and deep-vein thrombosis (Levine et al., 1996), have been safely treated at home with positive outcomes and quantifiable evidence of benefit in three predominant areas: clinical, financial, and customer satisfaction. Additionally there is an abundance of anecdotal patient and professional stories that support the home as a preferable treatment setting.

The overriding goal for home health care is to assist patients to attain their highest level of wellness. This global perspective necessitates the evaluation of opportunities and limitations associated with the patient's social support systems, physical living environment, financial means, and resources within the community, vistas that may be truncated when viewed only from the hospital window. Technology has all but eliminated the previous impediments to the "hospital-at-home," placing affordable, state-of-the-art patient care equipment and communication devices at the clinician's disposal. Patients and families consistently express a high degree of satisfaction with receiving care at home, encouraging compliance with the treatment regime.

The demand for home care as an appropriate venue will continue to evolve, driven by the increasing availability of technology and pharmaceuticals, more sophisticated consumers, and the escalating costs of health care (Campbell, 1998). Provider accountability will be substantially impacted by reimbursement and accreditation initiatives that will support only those providers who consistently demonstrate positive, cost-effective outcomes that compare favorably against traditional care. Is the shift of acute care from the hospital to home a good trend? Without a doubt!

REFERENCES

Campbell, L. (1998). *Home: The future of health care in America.* Kennett, MO: National HomeCare Database.

Levine, M., Gent, M., Hirsh, J., Leclerc, J., Anderson, D., & Weitz, J. (1996). A comparison of low-molecular-weight heparin administered primarily at home with unfractionated heparin administered in the hospital for proximal deep-vein thrombosis. *The New England Journal of Medicine, 334,* 677–681.

Talcott, J. A., Whalen, A., Clark, J., Rieker, P. P., & Finberg, R. (1994). Home antibiotic therapy for low-risk cancer patients with fever and neutropenia: A pilot study of 30 patients based on a validated prediction rule. *Journal of Clinical Oncology, 12,* 107–114.

The Balanced Budget Act of 1977, Pub. L. No. 105–33, 42 USC Section 4511, 4512 (1977).

Counterpoint

Bette K. Idemoto

While most nurses today have experienced the effects of health care reform, many have not considered the broader patient care issues associated with it. Early discharge, with the result of shifting acute care to the home, is one phenomenon arising from health care reform. The contrary view to early hospital discharge is presented to describe a set of difficulties associated with early discharge in assuring quality patient care while providing cost-effective care. Reasons for reconsideration of shifting acute care from the hospital to the home are: (1) lack of information about the total health care dollars spent for each particular patient population and/or diagnosis, including evaluating cost shifting from hospital to home care or skilled nursing facilities; (2) lack of information about the real outcomes of the total health/illness encounter, from diagnosis through return to health or management of chronic illness and death to helping to determine the quality of care; (3) need for increased nurse preparation to manage care across the continuum of care; (4) need for greater patient and family understanding of the realities of early discharge and increased family participation in post-hospital care; and (5) need for a better understanding of the impact of early discharge on the elderly, the very young, and other at-risk populations, including the poor, the uninsured, and the underinsured.

In an effort to decrease acute hospital costs, patients have been discharged earlier and earlier. The current health care schema, however, does not evaluate total health care dollars spent for episodes of care, nor is there significant knowledge of the costs associated with shifting care from hospital to home care agencies (HCA) or skilled nursing facilities (SNF) (Anderson & Helms, 1998; Gamblin, Hess, & Kenner, 1998). With early discharge, hospital length of stay (LOS) is decreased, yet the number of resulting patient days of SNF or HCA has not been adequately documented. Similarly, information about the extent of rehospitalization and emergency room visits associated with health episodes is just beginning to be systematically examined.

The difficulty with cost-shifting may soon be apparent with the cuts and changes in funding to the home care industry (Chang & Henry, 1999). The decreased level of funding and subsequent loss of home care assistance upon early discharge may result in increased readmissions and emergency room visits.

Next, before we can confidently say that the shift of acute care from the hospital to home is a positive trend, more information is needed about the quality of the outcomes associated with the total health/illness encounter. While some studies have shown positive effects of early discharge from acute hospitalization on selected populations, such as coronary artery bypass graft patients (Cowper, 1997; Riegel et al., 1996), other studies present contrary evidence. For example, studies of early maternal and neonatal discharge have indicated strong evidence of the need to increase the LOS for new mothers with uncomplicated deliveries (Malnory, 1997).

To meet the needs of an ever-changing health care field, nurses must be better prepared to handle expanding patient requirements in a shorter length of time spent in the acute setting (O'Halloran, 1997). Increased collaboration of care with other health care workers has become vital (Anderson, Nangle, & Alexander, 1997). To spend a limited time in the hospital means that nurses must be very experienced and efficient to be effective. Educating new nurses to maximize the days the patient has in the hospital is a huge challenge. Part of that responsibility lies in increasing the ability of bedside nurses to delegate care. Recognizing total patient needs and developing critical thinking skills in problem-solving often takes several years of experience at the bedside, and the profile of the nurses caring for patients often does not match this need.

Consumers also have a responsibility to understand the current health care market, including early discharge and requirements for increased family participation in post-hospital care. Most patients today remember when insurance paid more freely for hospital days and they are unprepared for the realities of managing acute illnesses in their homes. Some patients or families are unable or unwilling to cope with care needs. Even though efforts have been made by the media to articulate health care economic issues, most patients do not relate cost cutting to their personal situations. Attempts to discharge patients earlier are often met with resistance and resentment. The limited time to teach patients and families presents numerous challenges to an adequate preparation of patients for home care. Thus families often must bear the burden, frequently without adequate preparation. There also is increased concern that the elderly, who have more complex health and psychosocial problems and fewer resources (Bostrom, Crawford, Lazar, & Helmer, 1994; Espejo, Goudie, & Turpin, 1999; Grant, 1996; McCallum, Simons, Simons, Sadler, & Wilson, 1995; Schultz, Geary, Casey, & Fournier, 1997), may be the least able to learn adequate home care in the shortened time devoted to hospital-discharge teaching.

Last, the impact of the shift of acute care from the hospital to the home and the elderly, the very young, and other at-risk populations, including the poor, the uninsured and the underinsured, must be better understood. Examples of complex-care patients are those with heart failure, hip fractures, and strokes (Bours, Ketelaars, Frederiks, Abu-Saad, & Wouters, 1998; Grant, 1996; Intrator & Berg, 1998). Uncertainty regarding the amount of dollars available to assist the poor and uninsured, and the growing numbers of underinsured Americans, creates great concern for the future availability of resources to provide home care and SNFs for this population (McCallum et al., 1995).

Because the transitions that acute hospital care faces are not completed, nursing has an opportunity to help "fix" the cost-quality equation by awareness and action. Individual nurses at the bedside must know and articulate health care issues and participate in the process of growth and change. Organizationally, nurses must participate in policy development to create a health care environment that promotes quality within the cost restraints of today's health care market. The answer to shifting acute hospital care to home cannot be a positive "yes" until the issues presented here have been addressed.

REFERENCES

Anderson, J., Nangle, M., & Alexander, W. A. (1997). Cardiovascular outcome management and managed care contracting. *Critical Care Nursing Quarterly, 19*(4), 48–55.

Anderson, M. A., & Helms, L. B. (1998). Home care utilization by congestive heart failure patients: A pilot study. *Public Health Nursing, 15*(2), 146–162.

Bostrom, J., Crawford, L., Lazar, N., & Helmer, D. (1994). Learning needs of hospitalized and recently discharged patients. *Patient Education & Counseling, 23*(2), 83–89.

Bours, G. J. J., Ketelaars, C. A. J., Frederiks, C. M. A., Abu-Saad, H. H., & Wouters, E. M. (1998). The effects of aftercare on chronic patients and frail elderly patients when discharged from the hospital: A systematic review. *Journal of Advanced Nursing, 27,* 1076–1086.

Chang, W., & Henry, B. M. (1999). Methodologic principles of cost analyses in the nursing, medical and health services literature, 1990–1996. *Nursing Research, 48*(2), 94–104.

Cowper, P. (1997). The cost and cost effectiveness of coronary artery bypass graft surgery. In J. Talley (Ed.), *Cost effective diagnosis and treatment of coronary artery disease.* Baltimore: Williams & Watkins.

Espejo, A., Goudie, F., & Turpin, G. (1999). Hospital discharge into nursing home. *Aging & Mental Health, 3*(1), 69–78.

Gamblin, V., Hess, D. J., & Kenner, C. (1998). Early discharge from the NICU. *Journal of Pediatric Nursing: Nursing Care of Children and Families, 13*(5), 296–301.

Grant, J. S. (1996). Home care problems experienced by stroke survivors and their family caregivers. *Home Healthcare Nurse, 14*(11), 892–902.

Intrator, O., & Berg, K. (1998). Benefits of home health care after inpatient rehabilitation for hip fracture. *Archives of Physical Medicine and Rehabilitation, 79*(10), 1195–1199.

McCallum, J., Simons, L., Simons, J., Sadler, P., & Wilson, J. (1995). The continuum of care for older people: Increased concern about cost-shifting to community services. *Australian Health Review, 18*(2), 40–55.

Malnory, M. (1997). Maternal infant health care drives quality in managed care environment. *Journal of Nursing Care Quarterly, 11*(4), 9–26.

O'Halloran, V. E. (1997). Client education: Defining educational settings to improve client health teaching. *MEDSURG Nursing, 6*(3), 130–136.

Riegel, B., Gates, D. M., Gocka, I., Medina, L., Odell, C., Rich, M., & Finkel, J. S. (1996). Effectiveness of a program of early discharge of cardiac surgery patients. *Journal of Cardiovascular Nursing, 11*(1), 63–75.

Schultz, A. A., Geary, P. A., Casey, F., & Fournier, M. (1997). Joining education and service in exploring discharge needs. *Journal of Community Health Nursing, 14*(3), 141–153.

CHAPTER 5

Holistic Care: Is It Feasible in Today's Health Care Environment?

Point

Barbara M. Dossey

A frequently asked question is whether or not holistic care can be delivered in today's health care environment, and the answer is, yes, it can. Nurses must understand what holistic nursing is and what is involved in holistic care (Dossey, Keegan, & Guzzetta, 2000). Although the face of modern health care has changed, the essence of Florence Nightingale's message for holistic nursing and holistic care (Dossey, 2000) is the same. The American Holistic Nurses' Association (AHNA) Standards of Holistic Nursing Practice provide a working description of holistic nursing and clear guidelines for holistic care (AHNA, 2000):

> Holistic nursing embraces all nursing which has enhancement of healing the whole person from birth to death as its goal. Holistic nursing recognizes that there are two views regarding holism: that holism involves identifying the interrelationships of the bio-psycho-social-spiritual dimensions of the person, recognizing that the whole is greater than the sum of its parts; and that holism involves understanding the individual as a unitary whole in mutual process with the environment. Holistic nursing

Note: Originally published in *Nursing Leadership Forum*, Vol. 4, No. 4, 2000. New York: Springer Publishing Company.

responds to both views, believing that the goals of nursing can be achieved within either framework.

To facilitate the healing process and for nurses to become therapeutic partners with individuals, families, and communities, holistic nursing practice draws on nursing knowledge, theories, research, expertise, intuition, and creativity. Holistic nursing practice encourages peer review of professional practice in various clinical settings and integrates knowledge of current professional standards, laws, and regulations governing nursing practice.

Practicing holistic nursing requires nurses to integrate self-care in their lives. Self-responsibility leads the nurse to greater awareness of the interconnectedness with self, others, nature, and God/Life Force/Absolute/Transcendent. This awareness further enhances the nurses' understanding of all individuals and their relationships to the human and global community, and permits nurses to use this awareness to facilitate the healing process.

The AHNA Standards of Holistic Nursing Practice are used in conjunction with the American Nurses Association Standards of Practice and the specialty standards where holistic nurses practice. They contain five core values (see Table 5.1) that are followed by a description and standards of practice action statements. Holistic modalities draw on those derived from a number of explanatory models, of which biomedicine is one model. They reflect the diverse nursing activities in which holistic nurses are engaged and serve holistic nurses in personal life, clinical and private practice, education, research, and community service. Table 5.2 (p. 46) lists the most frequently used nursing interventions for holistic care.

To successfully integrate holistic care and holistic modalities, nurses must be aware of a fundamental principle that is involved with holistic care and holistic modalities, that is, the nurse facilitates the patient and significant others in their ability to be in the best state for healing to take place. Let me give two recent examples with my parents where nurses integrated holistic modalities with their technical work and also recognized that they were instruments of healing in this process. My 79-year-old mother had a knee replacement and on the third post-op day she became extremely agitated and confused as a result of a major aspect of post-surgical care—the use of technology

TABLE 5.1 Summary of Core Values of the American Holistic Nurses' Association

Core Value 1. Holistic Philosophy and Education

Holistic Philosophy: Holistic nurses develop and expand their conceptual framework and overall philosophy in the art and science of holistic nursing to model, practice, teach, and conduct research in the most effective manner possible.

Holistic Education: Holistic nurses acquire and maintain current knowledge and competency in holistic nursing practice.

Core Value 2. Holistic Ethics, Theories, and Research

Holistic Ethics: Holistic nurses hold to a professional ethic of caring and healing that seeks to preserve wholeness and dignity of self, students, colleagues, and the person who is receiving care in all practice settings, be it in health promotion, birthing centers, acute or chronic health care facilities, end-of-life care centers, or homes.

Holistic Nursing Theories: Holistic nurses recognize that holistic nursing theories provide the framework for all aspects of holistic nursing practice and transformational leadership.

Holistic Nursing and Related Research: Holistic nurses provide care and guidance to persons through nursing interventions and holistic therapies consistent with research findings and other sound evidence.

Core Value 3. Holistic Nurse Self Care

Holistic Nurse Self-Care: Holistic nurses engage in self-care and further develop their own personal awareness as being an instrument of healing to better serve self and others.

Core Value 4. Holistic Communication, Therapeutic Environment,
and Cultural Diversity

Holistic Communication: Holistic nurses engage in holistic communication to ensure that each person experiences the presence of the nurse as authentic and sincere; there is an atmosphere of shared humanness that includes a sense of connectedness and attention reflecting the individual's uniqueness.

Therapeutic Environment: Holistic nurses recognize that each person's environment includes everything that surrounds the individual, both the external and the internal (physical, mental, emotional, and spiritual) as well as patterns not yet understood.

TABLE 5.1 *(continued)*

Cultural Diversity: Holistic nurses recognize each person as a whole body-mind-spirit being and mutually create a plan of care consistent with cultural background, health beliefs, sexual orientation, values, and preferences.

Core Value 5. Holistic Caring Process

Assessment: Each person is assessed holistically using appropriate traditional and holistic methods while the uniqueness of the person is honored.

Patterns/Problems/Needs: Actual and potential patterns/problems/needs and life processes related to health, wellness, disease or illness which may or may not facilitate well-being are identified and prioritized.

Outcomes: Actual or potential patterns/problems/needs have appropriate outcomes specified.

Therapeutic Care Plan: A mutually created plan of care focuses on health promotion, recovery or restoration, or peaceful dying so that the person is as independent as possible.

Implementation: The mutual plan of holistic care is prioritized and holistic nursing interventions are implemented accordingly.

Evaluation: Responses to holistic care are regularly and systematically evaluated and the continuing holistic nature of the healing process is recognized and honored.

---

to ensure passive, continuous movement at the site of her knee replacement. When arriving to see Mom, I told Mom's nurse about her state, and she immediately addressed the situation with skill and compassion. She took Mom out of the electric device and assessed her pain level which was being managed properly. She next guided Mom in a relaxation and imagery exercise while integrating therapeutic touch for five minutes. Mom immediately fell asleep.

My father was diagnosed with non-Hodgkin's lymphoma and three months after his initial diagnosis and treatment with chemotherapy, he developed septic shock. Within five hours, in spite of superb critical care nursing and medical care, he died. It was a shock for all of us because just three months earlier, he appeared in excellent health, and as an avid golfer, he shot an 81 on his 81st birthday—a wonderful score! Daddy died from a bladder infection resulting from chemotherapy, not cancer.

The male nurse caring for my father was very tall and he had the critical care bed in the highest position while he worked. When Mom came into the room, he saw that she was barely 5 feet tall, and he immediately lowered the bed to let her get close and hug and kiss Daddy. Within the intensity of caring for my critically ill father, and the technical, critical care nursing, the nurse also integrated himself effectively as an instrument of healing by his sensitivity and therapeutic presence. His psychological and spiritual assessment of Mom's state made him aware of a very profound part of healing, doing an exquisite, very simple nursing act—lowering the bed for Mom. Because of this, our family has Daddy's last words that are part of the treasures that help us in our grieving process. Although my father was critical, he was alert enough to say to Mom in an irritated manner, "You can't believe what they are doing to me—all these tubes, oxygen, treatments. I wish they would just let me sleep!" Mom told him that it was to help him get well so that she could take him home. He pulled off his oxygen mask and said, "You think I'm going to get well?" Knowing how sick he was, and because the nurse had facilitated the physical environment to comfort Mom, she spoke from her heart and replied, "If not, I'll see you in heaven." She bent over, kissed Daddy and his final words to her were, "Okay, I'm so tired I'm going to turn over and take a little nap." Mom left the room, and as she did, my father immediately went into cardiac arrest and was unable to be resuscitated. The holistic care thereafter was also superb, a quiet room for family, friends, and the minister to gather together. The first physician to respond to the cardiac arrest code happened to be their neighbor whom they adored. After the nurse had removed all the tubes and equipment from the room, he came to ask if the family wanted to see Daddy again. Mother immediately said no. My brother and sister reported to me that the nurse paused with profound calmness and presence and said, "I just want you to know that he looks very peaceful." Mom experienced his words as a healing moment, and she returned to the bedside of the beloved man of her life for 56 years, accompanied by my brother and nephew who were with her at the time. My family and I will be forever grateful.

At the core of holistic care is spirituality and healing which encompasses a person's and/or family's values, meaning, and purpose in life. It reflects the human traits of caring, love, honesty, wisdom, and imagination, and it may reflect evidence of a higher power or higher

TABLE 5.2 Interventions Most Frequently Used In Holistic Nursing Practice[1]

Acupressure	Healing Presence	Play Therapy
Aromatherapy	Healing Touch Modalities	Prayer
Art Therapy	Holistic Self-Assessments	Reflexology
Biofeedback	Humor and Laughter	Relaxation Modalities
Cognitive Therapy	Journaling	Self-Care Interventions
Counseling[2]	Massage	Self-Reflection
Exercise and Movement	Meditation	Smoking Cessation
Goal-Setting and Contracts	Music and Sound Therapy	Therapeutic Touch
Guided Imagery	Nutrition Counseling	Weight Management

[1] See Dossey, B., Frisch, N., Forker, J., & Lavin, J. (1998).

[2] Used in situations such as addictions, death and grief, unhealthy environments, relationship issues, sexual abuse, spiritual needs, violence, support groups, wellness promotion, and lifestyle issues.

existence or a guiding spirit. The concept of spirit implies a quality of transcendence, a guiding force, or something outside the self and beyond the individual nurse or patient. This may or may not include the concept of organized religion which pertains to an organized group worship experience with other people who have a similar belief system. Spirit may suggest a purely mystical feeling or a flowing dynamic quality of unity that is ineffable. If one could clearly define the spirit, then it would no longer be the spirit. It is indefinable, yet it is a vital healing force profoundly felt by the individual and capable of affecting life and behavior.

Nurses are in a unique position to remember that they carry their healing with them at all times and are instruments of healing in every moment. Holistic care involves their sincere healing presence—a look, a smile, a hug, a few special actions or words allow their human spirit to become enfolded in one's being and the perceptions of meaning can make the difference between life and death.

To integrate holistic care, nurses must evolve their own personal healing process and increase reflections of healing in their personal lives such as with basic holistic modalities of relaxation, imagery, music, and touch (Dossey, Keegan, & Guzzetta, 1995). Nurses can become effective guides in a matter of minutes with holistic care and healing modalities, and truly become instruments in the healing process whether it is into health or the moment of death. As Florence Nightingale wrote about the importance of each nurse, she recognized the importance of one's own personal healing journey: ". . . and individual work . . . anything else is contrary to the whole realness of the work. Where am I, the individual in my utmost soul? What am I, the inner woman [man], called [I]?—That is the question . . ." (Dossey, 2000).

NOTE

For a complete copy of the AHNA Standards of Holistic Nursing Practice and information on American Holistic Nurses' Association (AHNA), Holistic Nursing Certification, and the Holistic Nursing Certification Examination contact: American Holistic Nurses' Association, P.O. Box 2130, 2733 Lakin Drive, Suite 2, Flagstaff, Arizona 86003-2130, (800) 278-AHNA, FAX (520) 526-2752.

REFERENCES

American Holistic Nurses' Association (AHNA). (2000). *Standards of Practice.* Flagstaff, AZ: Author.

Dossey, B. (2000). *Florence Nightingale: Mystic, visionary, healer* (p. 384). Springhouse, PA: Springhouse Corporation.

Dossey, B., Frisch, N., Forker, J., & Lavin, J. (1998). Evolving a blueprint for certification: Inventory of professional activities and knowledge of a holistic nurse. *Journal of Holistic Nursing, 16,* 33–56.

Dossey, B., Keegan, L., & Guzzetta, C. (1995). *The art of caring: Holistic healing using relaxation, imagery, music therapy, and touch.* Boulder, CO: Sounds True Audio Tapes.

Dossey, B., Keegan, L., & Guzzetta, C. (2000). *Holistic nursing: A handbook for practice* (3rd ed.). Gaithersburg, MD: Aspen Publishers, Inc.

Frisch, N., Dossey, B., Guzzetta, C., & Quinn, J. (2000). *The American Holistic Nurses' Association Standards of Holistic Nursing Practice: The integration of caring and healing.* Flagstaff, AZ: American Holistic Nurses' Association.

Counterpoint

Kathy Kolcaba

Today's health care environment is fraught with fast-paced change, scarcity of resources, and competition. Hospitals and agencies are struggling to retain contracts with large corporations and insurance companies. More and more, hospitals must demonstrate strength in aggregate outcomes such as patient satisfaction, few complications, adherence to critical pathways, etc. in order to maintain contracts with large groups of consumers (Corey-Lisle, Tarzian, Coben, & Trinkoff, 1999). These struggles for institutional viability render invisible the traditional mission of holistic nursing care (Benner, 1999).

Bumps in the road that nurses must negotiate are increased acuity and age of patients, shortened length of hospital stays, short staffing, and stringent criteria for home care reimbursement. Our sense of altruism keeps us on the road, but we are often poorly organized, tired, disillusioned, and fearful for the safety of our personal practice (Emler, 1999; Flipovich, 1999). We tend to view holistic care as "nice" but impossible under such conditions. A culture of defeatism is unable to promote conditions that facilitate holistic care.

A major detour that causes us to lose sight of the social mission of holistic care is that some nurses continue to align themselves with the medical model. This orientation is contradictory to our heritage (Fawcett, 1999). The goals of nursing practice and research have traditionally been to facilitate and explore person-environment interactions having to do with health (Benner, 1999; Fawcett, 1999; Schlotfeldt, 1981). From Nightingale (1860/1969), we inherited holism as our mandate with an emphasis on health. Through a prevention model, nurses teach health principles, enabling and empowering patients to achieve optimum function (LeVasseur, 1998; Salmon, 1999). Yet, the medical model continues to be copied and promoted through nursing diagnoses. Both medical and nursing diagnoses models focus on patients' problems which have narrow definitions and boundaries. The models, by their structure, look at parts rather than whole persons. Further, they fail to address health promotion in wider populations such as parishes, communities, and countries, and they fail to consider the environment as something to be manipulated to improve health (Schlotfeldt, 1981). These models have a disease (problem)-and-cure approach to the individual that dilutes the traditional foci of our discipline and obscures our distinct mission. Should this infatuation continue, holistic care cannot be valued or delivered.

SUSTENANCE FOR THE TRIP

In spite of economic forces that seem beyond our control, nurses have been doing a good job of "speaking" through patient satisfaction data collected by hospitals. These data show repeatedly that good nursing care is the chief predictor of good outcomes related to hospitalization (Lichtig, Knauf, & Milholland, 1999). Mass media have taken an interest in these data and are publicizing problems with patient safety associated with short and/or inexperienced staff, unlicensed assistive personnel, floating, mandatory overtime, and so forth (Flipovich, 1999; "20/20," 1999). Nurses have demonstrated that they make a difference for their patients and their institutions; however, articulating how they achieve these outcomes has been elusive.

Nurses must directly influence patient satisfaction by responding to what patients need from nurses. But what do patients need from nurses? "First and foremost, human beings—worldwide—want to be comforted and kept safe by nursing care" (Mallison, 1990). Patients report that they want "nurses who are concerned, attentive, and caring; who are competent and skilled; who communicate effectively with patients; who teach about condition, treatments, medications, and self-care; and who treat patients with respect" (Oermann, 1999, p. 51). Such attributes are entailed in holistic care and elevate holism as a primary goal for nursing and as a framework for achieving patient satisfaction.

Another source of strength for nurses is the public trust that our discipline has earned. In a recent Gallup pole of 1,000 persons, nursing was "Number 1" out of 100 professions for trustworthiness (Malone, 1999). This public trust is a source of grassroot support for stable and safe staffing, adequate wages, and improved working conditions for nurses—if nurses continue to give patients what they want and need, if patients continue to identify that their needs were met by nurses, and if nurses harness the public trust to support positive change. The current nursing shortage is an opportunity to voice solutions that would improve practice, to demonstrate our abilities to be managers as well as practitioners, and to unite for the greater good (Emler, 1999).

A BETTER ROAD SIGN

Holistic care is at the core of our identity as a discipline and at the heart of our support from the public; it is the traditional thread that unites us as nurses. Rather than give up on holistic care, we must remain focused on it under the most adverse (and in some cases perverse) societal forces that seek to weaken nursing. Therefore, the billboard question that generated this "counterpoint" perspective should not be "Is holistic care feasible in today's health care environment?" but rather "How can nurses deliver holistic care in today's health care environment?" For, if nurses lose sight of holism, their identity, common bond, and social mission will also be lost. Nurses will then be undifferentiated from other workers in the health care wilderness, leading to another cycle of downsizing and discouragement (Fawcett, 1999).

ESSENTIALS FOR THE JOURNEY INTO THE NEW MILLENNIUM

First, it is helpful to have a roadmap when trying to reach a goal, in this case a model or pattern for delivering holistic care. Some midrange theories offer a holistic roadmap for patient care, for example, Levine's "Conservation Theory" (1971), Kolcaba's "Comfort Theory" (1992), and Orlando's "Nurse-Patient Relationship" Model (1961/1990). Such models help organize our thinking and our work as nurses, so that nursing care is efficient, satisfying to patients and nurses, and, yes, holistic. It would be helpful if such models were routinely taught and applied in nursing education and made more available to practicing nurses.

Second, shifting from a focus on particular patient problems, entailed in the nursing diagnosis model, to a focus on patients' needs as whole persons seems a win-win strategy and one that has been advocated by many nurse leaders (Schlotfeldt, 1981; Fawcett, 1999). Patients have said they want holistic care from their nurses. A shift to recognizing and addressing what patients want from nurses, and doing it in an organized, professional way, will make nurses highly visible and indispensable in the health care arena.

Third, participating in conversations and demonstrations with administrators through bottom-up management will capitalize on the current power balance in favor of nurses brought about by the newest nursing shortage (Emler, 1999). Bottom-up management exists when workers vote on everything including whether a new coworker gets permanently hired and how the group schedules lunch breaks (Simon, 1999). In hospitals, nurses on each unit vote on and test models of scheduling, budgeting, assigning patient care, team-leading, rewarding workers, and so forth that work best in their setting. Models that "fit" and are cost-effective, morale-producing, and retention-demonstrating are maintained. In community nursing, similar models are advanced and tested by natural teams. By taking part in decision-making, nurses can create visions of and work toward workplaces that support holistic care.

Fourth, demonstrating through research that institutional outcomes are enhanced when holistic care is valued by administrators and allowed to be delivered is a necessary nursing strategy for the next millennium. Nightingale demonstrated through statistics that adverse outcomes were linked to infection caused by poor sanitation, lack of handwashing, contaminated water, and dirty dressings. She changed health care practice through research, thereby serving as a guide for our journey into the future. Our focus must be to address patients' holistic needs while demonstrating that improved outcomes from the patients' perspective also result in improved institutional outcomes.

Fifth, uniting for a common cause (nursing) through a common theme (holism) transcends differences in nursing such as entry levels for nursing practice, diverse roles nurses play, the myriad of educational backgrounds, and various styles of management. It is time to celebrate our commonalities, articulate what we know patients need and want from us, and demonstrate that we can deliver for the benefit of nursing and our institutions! It is time for proactive, positive, educated engagement in the mission of nursing.

REFERENCES

Benner, P. (1999). Claiming the wisdom and worth of clinical practice. *Nursing and Health Care Perspective, 29,* 312–320.

Corey-Lisle, P., Tarzian, A., Coben, M., & Trinkoff, A. (1999). Health care reform: Its effects on nurses. *Journal of Nursing Administration, 29*(3), 30–37.

Emler, J. (1999). Member sounds off about critical nursing shortage. *Ohio Nurses Review, 74*(10), 14.

Fawcett, J. (1999). The state of nursing science: Hallmarks of the 20th and 21st centuries. *Nursing Science Quarterly, 12,* 311–315.

Flipovich, C. (1999, August). Dealing with the issue of inadequate staffing. *Nursing, 99,* 54–56.

Kolcaba, K. (1992). A theory of holistic comfort for nursing. *Journal of Advanced Nursing, 19,* 1178–1184.

LeVasseur, J. (1998). Plato, Nightingale, and contemporary nursing. *Image: Journal of Nursing Scholarship, 30,* 281–285.

Levine, M. (1971). Holistic nursing. *Nursing Clinics of North America, 6,* 253–264.

Lichtig, L., Knauf, R., & Milholland, D. K. (1999). Some impacts of nursing on acute care hospital outcomes. *Journal of Nursing Administration, 29*(2), 25–33.

Mallison, M. (1990). Ninety years through nursing's lens. *American Journal of Nursing, 90*(10), 15.

Malone, B. (1999, November/ December). All I want for Christmas. . . . *The American Nurse,* 4.

Nightingale, F. (1969). *Notes on nursing: What it is, and what it is not.* New York: Dover Publications. (Original work published in 1860)

Oermann, M. (1999). Consumers' descriptions of quality health care. *Journal of Nursing Care Quality, 14*(1), 47–55.

Orlando, I. (1990). *The dynamic nurse-patient relationship.* New York: National League for Nursing. (Original work published in 1961)

Salmon, M. (1999). Thought on nursing: Where it has been and where it is going. *Nursing and Health Care Perspectives, 20,* 21–25.

Schlotfeldt, R. (1981, May). Nursing in the future. *Nursing Outlook, 29,* 295–301.

Simon, E. (1999, December 5). Bottom-up management no longer on the fringe. *The Plain Dealer,* p. 3–H.

20/20 (1999, November 26). New York: American Broadcasting Company.

CHAPTER 6

Telehealth: Can Nursing Values Be Preserved?

Point

Josette Jones

Interactive television, telepathology, e-mail, and teleconsults can be summed up in a single word: telehealth. Telehealth has been heralded as the next new wave in health care because of its potential to expand health care services beyond traditional geographic boundaries and give people in rural areas greater access to a broader range of care options. Patients who were hospitalized in the past are now treated in the comfort of their own homes. Nurses at a distant site, for example, can use telehealth to watch their patients take blood pressures, help them change a wound dressing, talk them through their medication regimens and explain symptoms.

As telehealth grows, and technical competence and speed of performance prevail, how will traditional core values of nursing subsist? Imagine for a moment the following scenario. Juanita Lopez, a 52-year-old, Spanish-speaking, insulin-dependent patient is discharged home 5 days after coronary artery graft bypass (CAGB) surgery. You are the home health nurse charged with the patient's follow-up in her rural home. Upon your initial assessment, you find infected incisions at both legs that require daily dressing changes. Additionally, her blood glucose is uncontrolled. As you plan on teaching her, you realize that your patient's understanding of her care is limited, and

Note: Originally published in *Nursing Leadership Forum*, Vol. 5, No. 2, 2000. New York: Springer Publishing Company.

that reinforcement is desirable for her to manage her care. Your knowledge of Spanish is limited, while Juanita's knowledge of English is minimal at best.

Your ability to provide effective and continuing care depends on your ability to find appropriate referrals, quick access to a Spanish interpreter, and patient-centered information in Spanish that answers questions about medication and treatment. The answer is telecommunication technology. Interactive TV or two-way video, attached to a computer in the patient's rural home, has the ability to access a Spanish-speaking nurse at a major medical center and send live videos of the patient while establishing an ongoing dialogue with the nurse about the patient's care. While the scenario may seem incredible, technology available today allows nurses to achieve this. Indeed, telecommunication technology not only enables the delivery of health care information and services for the patient's home, but also allows individualization and tailoring of health service activities to the care recipient's own situation and characteristics

Are these not the values most often cited as exemplifying the good, caring nurse? There is a timeless value of caring that links all nurses— caring in a committed way about the well-being of the people we serve. This fundamental value has helped nurses to move from the approach of "doing for" to the current focus on enabling and empowering (Salmon, 1999). Nursing theory, science, and intervention are inspired by and anchored to this core value.

Patients want their health care services custom tailored, preferably in the comfort of their homes. They desire health care services to be attendant to their specific disease and recovery trajectory, while at the same time being responsive to individual and family characteristics. It is possible with computer technology to assess cultural and educational background and beliefs and preferences and to address these differences with varying user computer interface designs (Jimison, 1997).

Also, patients seek answers to their questions at the time they are formulated. This is often after the nurse has left the face-to-face visit, not during the visit. E-mail link-ups between patients and nurses may help to answer patient questions in a timely manner. Patients also want access to more information. Nurses may direct them to World Wide Web (WWW) documents and community resources. Such resources provide patients and their family with confidence in their ability to engage in more self-directed care.

It is our attentiveness to patients' needs and preferences, effectiveness of treatments, efficiency in empowering patients, and the ability to appreciate and incorporate diversity that gives nurses' tasks and actions their meaning. Telehealth is bringing health care to patients' homes. Telehealth does not differ from or replace the more traditional health care delivery. Telehealth expands traditional health care services through telecommunication technology to areas that were previously underserved. Through telehealth, nurses have the ability to provide patients and families with care that is patient-centered, timely, and informative, with an emphasis on patient participation and an increased enticement to self-care.

REFERENCES

Jimison, H. B. (1997). Patient-specific interfaces to health and decision-making information. In R. L. Street, W. R. Gold, & T. Manning (Eds.), *Health promotion and interactive technology: Theoretical applications and future directions.* Mahwah, NJ: Lawrence Erlbaum.

Salmon, M. E. (1999). Thoughts on nursing: Where it has been and where it is going. *Nursing and Health Care Perspectives, 20*(1), 20–25.

Counterpoint

Shirley M. Moore

Although computers are often associated with the business functions of health care delivery (Behrend, 1994) and decision support for professionals (Paperny, Aono, Lehman, Hamar, & Risser, 1990), their use to deliver patient care has progressed slowly. More recently, however, common nursing functions, previously accomplished in face-to-face interactions, are beginning to be done using computer communications. Integrating the "high touch" values commonly associated with nursing care into the design of computerized nursing care delivery systems is a challenge that must be met if the widespread use of technology-mediated care is to be realized.

Over the past 50 years nurses have increasingly used technology to support the care they provide. The use of technology in health care has progressed to the point where home care nurses frequently use machines, such as ventilators, in people's homes. It has been suggested that modern nursing is deeply connected to technology development (Barnard, 1999). Nurses' attitudes toward computers, however, tend to indicate that they are undecided about computer technology. In a survey of hospital nurses, McConnell and colleagues (1989) found that, although nurses thought that the use of computers improved the quality of patient care, they also believed that their use dehumanized the care. It should be noted that one half of the nurses surveyed had no experience with computers. Another view dominant in the nursing literature is that nurses are the patient's bridge from the impersonal, technologic world to the humanistic world (McConnell, 1998). This technologic-humanistic dualistic philosophical view has fostered nurses' fears about the increase of technical quality at the expense of humanness. Thus, as a group, nurses have been reticent to embrace computer-mediated care.

Nurses are socialized to a set of values in their professional education and practice. Nursing values of (a) individualizing care, (b) fostering self-care, (c) maintaining caring interpersonal relationships, (d) supporting patient autonomy, and (e) providing collaborative care must be considered in the design and implementation of electronic tools to support nursing care. Although the successful delivery of health care presumes a certain degree of standardization of treatments and interventions, nursing values reinforce modifying care away from the "one size fits all" model. Nursing care focuses on tailoring care to the unique needs of patients and their families. Fostering self-care refers to nurses' support and education of patients to engage in activities that are health-promoting.

Basic to nursing values is the helping relationships in which nurses engage with their patients (Morse, Solberg, & Neander, 1990). This relationship progresses over time as the nurse interacts with her patients to manage health problems by building trust through genuine caring and encouraging patients to share their thoughts and feelings. Through intimate interpersonal relationships, nurses conduct activities aimed at restoring physical, emotional, spiritual, and social well-being. Additionally, nurses have historically fostered patient autonomy by supporting patients' rights to make decisions about their health. Nurses also value collaboration with other health care professionals to plan care. While nursing will always require some face-to-face interaction (e.g., bathing patients, physical examinations), many nursing caregiver functions are amenable to computer mediation, such as symptom monitoring, the provision of information, assistance with decision-making, and providing emotional support. Computer-mediated nursing care delivery systems represent a new environment for therapeutic nurse-patient relationships. Therefore, as electronic health care delivery systems are developed, we must be mindful of professional nursing values and essential nursing functional roles.

Clinical interventions using computers require nurses to have an understanding of how computer technology affects client participation, communication, relationship development, and group norms, including both social and computer behavior (Moore, 1997). Challenges of computer communications that affect the nursing system of care include: the lack of physical presence of clients, diffuse time referents, asynchronous communication, and the necessity to teach clients to use the technology. The absence of face-to-face visual cues requires nurses to rely on a new set of cues, many of which differ from those of clinical encounters involving face-to-face or voice communication. Developing and maintaining relationships are goals of any therapeutic clinical encounter. Rapport and trust can be developed between the nurse and clients through the use of standard protocols for computer "introductions" among participating parties, encouragement of the use of a conversational tone in messages posted on the system, and nurse modeling of emotional expressions in messages.

The nurse's role as educator has expanded with the increased use of Web-based health care information by patients. Nurses must learn to critically analyze website content, source of content, quality of content, and intended audience. When patients present information downloaded from the Internet, nurses must be prepared to analyze the information for accuracy and applicability and advise patients about the proper use of Web-based health care resources and current treatment interventions. Teaching patients how to use search engines, bookmark favorite websites, and access health-related support groups are examples of patient education skills nurses soon will be providing on a daily basis. Nurses are also beginning to develop Web pages containing health information for clients. This is an important role for nurses since they are knowledgeable about how to tailor information to appropriate reading levels, cultural aspects, and developmental needs of patients.

Over the past 10 years, experiences in the design and testing of electronic nursing care delivery systems have provided insights about the potential impact of electronic care delivery systems on the work of nurses. Nurses are learning about the ideal "client load" that can be reasonably managed electronically by a nurse or health care team, how much electronic client contact should be done individually or in groups, the extent to which clients' families can be involved, and the correct balance between the amount of work done with clients on-line and using other forms of communication, i.e., telephone, writing, or face-to-face contacts. Nurses are also learning about design features that are important to patients and nurses.

Technology is an important factor in the evolution of nursing practice and the experience of nursing (Barnard, 1996). A technologic-humanistic dualism does not have to exist in technology-mediated nursing care. Challenges to the humanistic aspects of nursing (maintaining "high touch" in a "high tech" system) can be sufficiently managed only if computerized nursing care delivery systems include design features mindful of professional nursing values.

REFERENCES

Barnard, A. (1996). Technology and nursing: An anatomy of definition. *International Journal of Nursing Studies, 33*, 433–441.

Barnard, A. (1999). Nursing and the primacy of technological progress. *International Journal of Nursing Studies, 36*, 435–442.

Behrend, S. W. (1994). Documentation in the ambulatory setting. *Seminars in Oncological Nursing, 10*, 264–280.

McConnell, E. A. (1998). The coalescence of technology and humanism in nursing practice: It doesn't just happen and it doesn't come easily. *Holistic Nursing Practice, 12*, 23–30.

McConnell, E. A., O'Shea, S. S., & Kirchhoff, K. T. (1989). RN attitudes toward computers. *Nursing Management, 20*, 36–40.

Moore, S. M. (1997). Computer networks as environments for care: Dynamics of the clinical encounter. In P. Brennan, S. Schneider, & E. Tornquist (Eds.), *Community health care information networks* (pp. 287–297). New York: Springer-Verlag.

Morse, J., Solberg, S., & Neander, W. (1990). Concepts of caring and caring as a concept. *Advances in Nursing Science, 13*(1), 1.

Paperny, D. M., Aono, J. Y., Lehman, R. M., Hamar, S. L., & Risser, J. (1990). Computer-assisted detection and intervention in adolescent high-risk health behaviors. *Journal of Pediatrics, 116*, 456–462.

CHAPTER 7

Building a Better Mousetrap: The Upside of Downsizing

Perspectives From Education

Cynthia Caroselli

Health care providers throughout the nation are currently experiencing what is arguably the most significant upheaval in the history of health care in this country. While many people are concerned with reimbursement issues, skill mix modifications, and mergers and acquisitions, the overwhelming majority of efforts are related to what is often referred to as "the R word"—restructuring. Also known as redesign, reorganization, or in its most dreaded form, downsizing, this phenomenon is widely regarded as health care's most distressing nightmare. Redesign inspires as much confusion as it does fear; many assume that redesign is synonymous with downsizing. Most assume that it has only undesirable consequences. Two things are abundantly clear: One, this upheaval will continue for the foreseeable future, and two, we must completely change the way in which we perform our work.

For nurses in practice environments, redesign can be seen as an opportunity for reinvention. While it may take some mental gymnastics to view redesign as an opportunity, it does present leaders in these areas with the opportunity to make major changes that can ensure that a nursing perspective guides reinvention.

Note: Originally published in *Nursing Leadership Forum*, Vol. 2, No. 2, 1996. New York: Springer Publishing Company.

For those in nursing education, however, redesign represents more than an opportunity. Redesign mandates that nursing education change the way in which it carries out its mission, but the mandate is much larger than this. The daunting task that nursing education faces is that of preparing practitioners at all levels with the skills that will enable them to survive these tumultuous times as well as with skills that will allow them to move through the next millennium with a tolerance for ambiguity, a facility for cost management, and finely honed skills for adding value and quality to the services they provide, irrespective of role or setting. A challenging agenda indeed.

Change can no longer occur in piecemeal fashion, simply adding to an already overloaded curriculum. It is critical that both product and process be redesigned. Change must occur in the fundamental processes of education, so that the product, the graduate, is significantly different from that of years past.

Redesign must be, in the words of Hammer and Champy (1993), fundamental, radical, and dramatic. While past efforts at improvement may have centered on incremental gains based on doing more and doing it better (Tonges, 1992), this approach is no longer helpful. Redesign means embarking on a radical departure from the norm, creating new methods and structures, with resultant changes in processes, cultures, services, and behaviors for the sole purpose of survival in a threatened environment (Flarey, 1995). For nursing education, this means the abandonment of a long tradition of processes and traditions that many see as sacred.

The process of education, long categorized into rigid time frames, must loosen and become more adaptable to the changing needs and competing demands of a student body that is consistently older, working longer hours, and responsible for young children and aging parents. To address the needs of this changed student body at all levels of education, we must take our process apart and recombine its elements into more adaptable systems. Efforts in place for weekend and evening classes and clinical placements must continue, but at a more rapid pace. Provision of day care for dependent children and the elderly could form the basis of clinical practica while addressing student issues that impede learning, on virtually a budget-neutral basis.

A major component of successful redesign efforts is the envisioning of outcomes from the start (Flarey, 1995). This is a difficult task for educators who are struggling with the seemingly oppositional outcomes of preparing students for licensure and/or certification exams that are focused on current-day practice while also preparing graduates for an uncertain environment. While outcomes may be difficult to determine in terms of specific knowledge bases that will be relevant 10 years hence, central concepts and values are somewhat easier to determine. These frameworks are consistent with nursing's core values of caring, humanistic service to patients, families, and communities. Beliefs about respect for the individual's cultural, spiritual, sexual, intellectual, emotional, and physical needs remain central, but should be broadened to apply to emerging constituencies and structures.

Students at all levels need to understand that health care is a product and a service, not a place. Thinking about critical care as occurring outside of the ICU, surgical procedures performed in community settings, or childbirth in the home encourages "out of the box" thinking that can lead to new approaches to care delivery or to new solutions to old problems. While it is possible to teach practicing nurses these concepts, it is more practical to introduce students to this kind of critical thinking early in their educational experiences. It can ease the tension of reality shock (Kramer & Schmalenberg, 1993) and reflects the widespread belief that critical thinking is one of the most useful skills for the health care delivery system of the future (National League for Nursing, 1991).

Another critical knowledge base relates to finance. Regardless of setting or role, cost management is no longer the sole responsibility of the finance department; managers and care providers alike must apply financial skills to care organization and delivery (Fralic & Flarey, 1995). This is part of a larger issue, namely, the preparation of nurses for what can be termed organizational citizenship. Being a fully functional, organizational citizen means recognizing that nursing is part of a larger whole, that adding value to services provided to clients will do much to ensure organizational survival (Patterson, 1992) and that cost containment will remain an imperative for all areas of health care. The notion of the seamless health care environment, frequently mentioned as a desirable goal, must be reified in actual practice so that managers and care providers see collaboration as the means to the end of user-friendly services. This is in contrast with the long established tradition of turf wars among the various health care disciplines; such infighting will not only result in fragmented care for the client but will also virtually assure that the health care organization will die in a blaze of controversy. Thus, conflict negotiation and collaboration must be incorporated into curricula for all types of role-specific education. Getting to YES (Fisher, Ury, & Patton, 1991) must be seen as valuable for service delivery as well as organizational viability.

Educators who prepare students for staff nurse roles, whether in generic or completion programs, should understand clearly the realities of the practice arena, both as currently configured and as projected for the future. Generally, students must understand that change will be a fact of their professional lives for the duration of their careers. Appreciation of the opportunities presented by change will help them to cope with the accompanying stresses. This could be operationalized, for instance, by honing the students' skills in assessment of organizational culture, recognizing shifts in the cultural paradigm, and formulating a response that allows the graduate to become an organizational hero (Caroselli, 1992).

A valuable adjunct for any career is the acquisition of mentors who can alert the mentee to opportunities as well as to developmental needs (Kerfoot, 1995). Specifics related to finding and utilizing a mentor should become part of the socialization of the student to the professional role.

Students must be assisted to develop long-term career goals that will allow them to enjoy a diverse career. While faculty have traditionally cautioned graduates to focus on narrowing their interests to a particular role or practice area, it is probably wiser to encourage students to develop a broad portfolio of skills in addition to increasing the depth of their knowledge bases related to a specific patient population. For instance, while a student may have a strong interest in critical care, the graduate's long-term marketability would be enhanced by home health skills and experience, since critical care is now being delivered in many areas outside the confines of the acute care hospital.

As health care moves toward the paperless environment, and in light of the vast amount of data collection that has become integral to care, electronic communication skills are considered essential for staff nurse practice (AONE, 1995). Basics such as searching electronic data bases, e-mail correspondence, Web searching, and word processing should be incorporated into class assignments so that students are prepared upon graduation to use information systems and able to function as members of special project teams (Sovie, 1990).

Shared governance has become a common phenomenon in health

care organizations, and has resulted in a stronger voice for the staff nurse, with an actual role in the regulation of nursing practice. Because this requires the assumption of some duties traditionally thought of as managerial, staff must acquire broadened business and collaborative skills (Dienemann & Gessner, 1992) in order to function appropriately in what must be seen as an expansion of the staff nurse role. Thus, content to develop these skills must be included in undergraduate curricula as preparation for beginning practice.

Nursing managers and administrators feel particularly beleaguered in the stressful environment of restructuring, and while some stress is directly attributable to the obvious tumult of redesign, it can be posited that the educational preparation of nurse managers has not adequately addressed their actual needs. Changes in health care as an industry have forced nursing administrators to assume a broader scope of responsibilities and to implement programs that provide high-quality, cost-effective care delivered by an increasingly productive nursing staff (Scalzi & Wilson, 1990). This is reflected in the growing phenomenon of nurse managers assuming responsibility for more than one unit and nurse executives overseeing the entire realm of patient services, not simply the department of nursing. Similarly, nurse executives are required to interpret and sell programs in terms of what is beneficial for the entire organization, not just for nursing (Tonges, 1992). Simply put, this requires leading across cultural, functional, and departmental boundaries, as well as tolerating ambiguity and perpetual change (AONE, 1995).

Educational implications for administrators are clear. A strong foundation in finance, marketing, policy analysis, and information management is essential (Scalzi & Wilson, 1990). Project management skills are also important (Kerfoot, 1995), since administrators will continue to be involved in matrix arrangements that will structure work teams temporarily around specific assignments. And while staff nurses need to be able to assess the culture of an organization, administrators need to have the skills necessary to create and mold a culture that will facilitate a patient-driven, user-friendly environment. Clearly, nursing theory is the core of such efforts and forms the value system from which decisions are made.

Many nurses are enrolled in advanced practice programs, preparing to assume positions as nurse practitioners, clinical nurse specialists, nurse midwives, or nurse anesthetists. While it can be assumed that these roles will continue to grow in number and in scope over the foreseeable future, it is important that nurses consider these roles within the scope of the mission of the organization. While many nurses choose these roles based upon the care of a particular patient population or on the performance of specific activities, long-term marketability is founded on service to the organization as a whole. For instance, many advanced practice nurses find themselves functioning as case managers and developing care protocols (Guiliano & Poirier, 1991), coalescing the various components and disciplines available in an organization for the provision of seamless care. Nursing theory is an essential prerequisite as is the ability to negotiate, collaborate, and "nurse the system." While this may not have been the initial attraction to the role, advanced practice nurses equipped with these skills will find that they can make a greater impact on patient care by incorporating these skills into their repertoires.

Nurse educators have seen their roles in many settings evolve. Staff development educators have perhaps felt the sting of restructuring most acutely, given the downsizing that many organizations have implemented in these departments. In addition, the introduction of greater numbers of unlicensed assistive personnel (UAP) (Flarey, 1995) has changed the skill mix in virtually every health care facility. Since these roles are designed to be assistive to the professional nurse, it is entirely appropriate that nurse educators, however, provide UAP training. Many programs that prepare nurse educators, however, utilize a model that is grounded in teaching nursing students, who constitute a vastly different group of learners than UAP. Thus, nurse educator preparation should include a greater emphasis on adult learning theory applied to various levels of learner literacy, a deeper understanding of cultural diversity, and a greater facility for creating electronic learning resources, such as multimedia programs. In addition, since consumers have become more sophisticated and now demand greater information and ask more questions, nurse educators need to be prepared to ask the questions: Who is the constituency? What do they need? What is the most appropriate vehicle for addressing these needs? In addition to sophisticated electronic learning skills, it may be appropriate to include epidemiological content such as community assessment into nurse educator curricula.

Doctoral students are often seen as "the cream of the crop" engaged in the generation of new knowledge, and thus by definition on the "cutting edge." Yet, restructuring of health care should figure in these programs as well. Doctoral education should incorporate policy analysis so that graduates will be prepared to shape a national research agenda and to influence funding priorities based on a strong nursing conceptual basis. Indeed, theory development and application should begin at the doctoral level since redesign efforts should begin with the specification and definition of a theoretical model (Flarey, 1995).

While this paper has delineated a number of ways in which nursing education must be redesigned in light of health care restructuring, and while the ideas set forth are challenging and require a Herculean effort, it is important to recognize that these challenges bring with them enormous opportunity. The product of these efforts, the graduate, will be better prepared to deal with current and future challenges, and may in fact be better prepared than other members of the health care delivery team. Further, restructuring will allow graduates to be better prepared for long-term marketability and a career that can evolve through a future of uncertainty. So, while restructuring is a choice that few of us would have made willingly, it is not totally grim. Redesign can result in a situation in which we can rectify some of the ills from which the educational system has been suffering. The possibilities can be exciting, and the results could be enriching.

REFERENCES

AONE (1995). *The impact of organizational redesign on nurse executive leadership* (Part II). Irving, TX: VHA, Inc.

Caroselli, C. (1992). Assessment of organizational culture: A tool for professional success. *Orthopaedic Nursing, 11*(3), 57–63.

Dienemann, J., & Gessner, T. (1992). Restructuring nursing care delivery systems. *Nursing Economics, 10*(4), 253–310.

Fisher, R., Ury, W., & Patton, B. (1991). *Getting to yes: Negotiating an agreement without giving in.* Boston: Houghton Mifflin Co.

Flarey, D. L. (Ed.). (1995). *Redesigning nursing care delivery: Tranforming our future.* Philadelphia: J.B. Lippincott.

Fralic, M.F., & Flarey, D.L. (1995). Integrating quality into care delivery systems redesign. In D.L. Flarey (Ed.), *Redesigning nurs-*

ing care delivery: Transforming our future (p. 35). Philadelphia: J.B. Lippincott.

Giuliano, K. K., & Poirier, C.E. (1991). Nursing case management: Critical pathways to desirable outcomes. *Nursing Management, 22*(3), 52–55.

Hammer, M., & Champy, J. (1993). *Reengineering the corporation: A manifesto for business revolution.* New York: HarperBusiness.

Kerfoot, K. (1995). Managing your career as a contingent worker: The nurse manager's challenge. *Nursing Economics, 13*(3), 178–180.

Kramer, M., & Schmalenberg, C. (1993). Learning from success: Autonomy and empowerment. *Nursing Management, 25*(5), 58–64.

National League for Nursing. (1991). *Nursing data source 1991: Leaders in the making: Graduate education in nursing.* New York: NLN Pub. No. 19–2422.

Patterson, C. (1992). The economic value of nursing. *Nursing Economics, 10*(3), 193–204.

Scalzi, C. C., & Wilson, D. L. (1990). Empirically based recommendations for content of graduate nursing administration programs. *Nursing and Health Care, 11*(10), 522–525.

Sovie, M. D. (1990). Redesigning our future: Whose responsibility is it? *Nursing Economics, 8*(1), 21–26.

Tonges, M.C. (1992). Work designs: Sociotechnical systems for patient care delivery. *Nursing Management, 23*(1), 27–31.

Perspectives From Practice

Joanne Baggerly

While the number of nurses in inpatient settings will likely continue to be adjusted to align with declining patient census, the need for professional nursing judgment and skills in the clinical setting is even greater. The reality of "downsizing" has generated a great deal of angst. Emotional responses, such as fear and/or anger, have led some to employ strategies that appear to be somewhat reactionary in nature. The "rhetoric" of encouraging patients to ask about whether a nurse will be caring for them or their loved one, for example, may raise the consciousness of consumers, but will do little to demonstrate the difference a nurse can make and is likely to widen the gulf between various nursing groups and nurse administrators who acutely feel the burden of decisions that must be made in response to environmental demands. On the other hand, there is certainly abundant evidence of nursing's ability to develop clinically sound and innovative approaches to positively impact outcomes (Brooten et al., 1986), as well as creatively respond to the demands of capitation (Lowe, 1996). Suggestions and direction for improving practice, education, and research to correspond with externally imposed changes are apparent (Caroselli, 1992; Fagin, 1996). In addition to these constructive efforts and recommendations, there is a pragmatic need to view downsizing as an occasion to not only redesign care delivery systems, but to rethink the types of information necessary to demonstrate the value of nursing.

Nurse leaders in the practice arena need to seize opportunities to make "invisible" aspects of practice more obvious. This requires political savvy and an expansion of the view of our "customer" from clients to include administrators and third party payers. The skill of "perspective taking" and identification of client needs that is part of the basic repertoire of nurse leaders in the clinical setting must be expanded to include an understanding of what is valuable to these "customers." Clinical concerns must be linked to mutual concerns and the interests of all of these groups. The ability to manage care problems and influence outcomes represents one such area of common concern. Our collective efforts need to clearly focus on demonstrating contributions to cost-effective, efficient patient care outcomes.

Advanced clinical knowledge and preparation must be supplemented with new skills, particularly in the areas of information management. Program evaluation and epidemiological methods offer the means to objectively quantify the volume of common patient risks and problems managed by nurses. Such information provides clinically driven rationale to justify programs, establish priorities, and a starting point to evaluate the impact on outcomes. This shift in emphasis will position nurse leaders to respond more proactively to changes in the practice setting and demonstrate the impact of nursing on outcomes of care, but will necessitate familiarity with and participation in the development of databases which can be used to gather information for analysis and identification of outcomes associated with various programs or aspects of care.

Much of the outcome information currently available is devoid of data that reflect nursing contributions to the cost-effective management of patient populations. Fiscal, risk management, performance and outcome improvement, and infection control data have provided the majority of outcome information available to clinicians. But such data are without context. Even when linked to a diagnosis, medical intensity and other variables which affect outcomes are absent, thus precluding transformation of the data into information which is essential for meaningful analysis. The traditional performance and outcome improvement approach, for example, has been to establish "thresholds," and when cross-sectional data indicate that the threshold has been surpassed, investigation and action must occur. While this effort promotes accountability and stimulates further investigation, developing meaningful practice actions from the data alone is difficult, if not impossible. An increase or decrease in some rate from one time period to another may really reflect changes in the population that are outside the control of practitioners, such as severity, comorbidities, or prognosis. A rate in a given time period may be below the threshold, yet include events in some patients that would reflect a poor outcome or conversely reflect acceptable outcomes despite higher than targeted thresholds. To illustrate this point, consider a stroke patient who did not achieve continence by discharge. Without information regarding the stroke type and severity, stage of recovery within the context of the disease trajectory, or other variables known to be associated with improvement, no meaningful conclusion can be drawn about the appropriateness of this outcome.

Outcome databases for specific patient populations that include acuity, medical intensity, and other variables will enhance the evaluation of cost and efficacy of care. Outcomes must be established that include consideration of the recovery potential and expected progress toward that outcome. The potential for recovery and estimated trajectory for the problem must drive interventions and resources to be allocated. Population-specific care maps or pathways, protocols, and algorithms will decrease variability and assist nurses in this task.

Nursing can play a role in providing the clinical link that has been missing by forming new alliances with those involved with existing financial databases and by strengthening alliances with physicians to assure that clinical variables that influence outcomes are considered. Extending the traditional conception of outcomes to include those related to nurse-managed problems will provide a better picture of cost and value. Nursing acuity data can contribute another perspective to this picture as well. Comparisons of price and value in various settings relative to outcomes will be enhanced.

Given the current "continuum of care" concept, we need to develop measures that will reflect the occurrence and resolution of problems throughout the illness/disease trajectory, as well as identify expected outcomes for speck phases. Changes, such as early discharge from acute care, have led to a shift in the burden of care to the community or other settings. While it is often stated that this has occurred without adverse consequences, it is more accurate to state that many of the specific implications of this shift have not been captured. Variables other than fiscal or medical complication rates have not been measured, thus important consequences have not been articulated. Epidemiological methods can be very helpful in quantifying problems, establishing priorities, and providing baseline measurements for evaluation of the strategies put in place to manage problems. Consideration of one aspect of care, the prevalence and incidence of pressure sores, will illustrate this point. Anecdotal information from home care nurses indicates that there has been an increase in the number of patients admitted with pressure sores. In response to a similar concern in our rehabilitation setting, we initiated a prevalence and incidence study that revealed that 23% of the patients were being admitted with a pressure sore and 45% were at risk for the development of one. The information was invaluable to the nurse executive in budgeting, and justifying the resources for program development and a system for tracking the outcomes for pressure sores and pressure-sore risk was developed. Had we not seized the opportunity, the implications for patient outcomes would not be identified and the value of nursing assessment and intervention relative to both management and prevention would remain invisible. Additionally, nursing knowledge regarding extent and duration of the problem, at least for the particular setting and population, would not have been uncovered.

Prevalence and incidence data are essential for evaluation of prevention programs (Allcock, Wharrad, & Nicolson, 1994). Prevalence data describe the magnitude of a problem, while incidence data are necessary to evaluate the effectiveness of prevention and/or education programs. Incidence data are particularly valuable in our setting because we cannot control whether patients are admitted with a pressure sore or at risk for development of one, but we can develop programs aimed at prevention and evaluate the effectiveness by examining incidence data. Descriptive knowledge of problems can also provide the groundwork for the development of better research questions.

Nurses have traditionally prided themselves on the ability to manage patient care problems, but have done this "silently." Opportunities to make nursing actions more visible must be recognized to ensure that the value of nursing and the need for nursing intervention are articulated. Because patient risks and problems require nursing skill and assessment, as patients continue to move through the "continuum of care," it is important to learn more about the duration of risks and problems specific to each phase to ensure that outcomes are maintained. While the current emphasis is on the costs associated with providing care in various settings, ultimately outcome data for identified patient problems will be necessary. Only with such information can the "value" and costs of care provided in various settings in terms of the outcomes for patients be identified.

From a practice perspective, descriptive data on the volume, duration, and outcome for various risks and problems will contribute to nursing knowledge. Epidemiological methods provide an approach for identifying the volume and types of problems experienced by patients and managed by nurses. As we "redesign" systems of care, this information will be invaluable in articulating the requirements for professional nursing assessment and intervention. Finally, the availability of such information provides feedback and allows clinicians to be actively engaged in the process of investigating phenomena in the practice arena.

Of course there is much more to nursing than can be measured, but measurement is what is valued and respected. We must become more adept at employing epidemiological methods to quantify problems, establish priorities, and evaluate the effectiveness of restructuring and redesign. In so doing we will be able to keep more of the unmeasurable and immeasurable essence of nursing.

REFERENCES

Allcock, N., Wharrad, H., & Nicolson, A. (1994). Interpretation of pressure-sore prevalence. *Journal of Advanced Nursing, 26,* 37–45.

Brooten, D., Kumar, S., Brown, L., Butts, P., Finkeler, S. A., Bakewell-Sachs, S., Gibbons, A., & DeLivoria-Papadopoulos, M. (1986). A randomized clinical trial of early hospital discharge and home follow up of very low birthweight infants. *New England Journal of Medicine, 315*(15), 934–939.

Caroselli, C. (1992). Assessment of organizational culture: A tool for professional success. *Orthopaedic Nursing, 11*(3), 57–63.

Fagin, C. M. (1996). Executive leadership improving nursing practice, education, and research. *Journal of Nursing Administration, 26*(3), 30–37.

Lowe, A. (1996). Reducing variation in patient care: Nursing responds to capitation. *Journal of Nursing Administration, 26*(1), 14–20.

CHAPTER 8

Sharing the Vision: The Views From Nursing Management and Staff

The View From Nursing Management

Tara A. Cortes

In today's health care environment the conceptualization and understanding of one's role in an organization is more important than ever before. With shrinking resources the need for every health care professional to recognize the importance of his/her contribution to an organization's mission is paramount to the success of the organization.

Nurses continue to comprise the largest percentage of caregivers in organized health care systems. The ability of professional nurses, from beginning practitioners to the most advanced and specialized nurse practitioner, to be accountable and responsible is essential to the continuing autonomy and viability of the profession (Porter-O'Grady, 1994). A staff nurse needs minimally to be able to independently execute the nursing process in a complex environment that has no boundaries. Additionally, this nurse needs to be able to manage resources in a cost-effective manner.

The days of enormous nursing budgets and major recruitment efforts in nursing by hospitals are over. There are nursing positions available, but nursing administrators want the "brightest and the best"

Note: Originally published in *Nursing Leadership Forum*, Vol. 2, No. 4, 1996. New York: Springer Publishing Company.

nurses because with shrinking resources nurses must be accountable for their practice in a highly productive manner. For this reason many nursing administrators tend to avoid hiring new graduates and seek more experienced nurses who can enter any health care system and produce the workload of a calculated, full-time employee (FTE) in as short a period of time as possible. With fewer nurse positions available, many nurse administrators simply cannot afford to fill a position with a nurse who cannot assume full responsibility for the nurse role and who consumes the time of other nurse resources in the forms of guidance, mentoring, and assistance in decision-making.

The new graduate, however, is not the only nurse who does not assume full responsibility and accountability in professional practice. There are also nurses who have worked in health care for a varied number of years and have never assimilated professionalism into their practice. These nurses never seem to be willing to take responsibility for decision-making, to be accountable for their job without supervisory follow-up, or to reach out of the comfort of their daily routine to design or even think about new ways of practice that could enhance the institution's ability to fulfill its missions and goals. These nurses leave those professional and visionary responsibilities to those nurse professionals who do, fortunately, make up the majority of hospital staffs. Without every nurse assuming full accountability for practice, however, the institution falls short of its potential in productivity.

The nursing administrator is faced with the challenge of recruiting, developing, maintaining, and retaining a staff which shares the philosophy, vision, and goals of the organization and fulfills its role with commitment and enthusiasm. This is only possible when the staff recognizes that what they do is vital to the success of the organization. If the caregivers and others who actually provide patient care do not represent the values of the institution, all the best laid plans will not save it from decline in a capitated, consumer-driven health care system (Evans, Aubrey, Hawkins, Curley, & Porter-O'Grady, 1995). This means that the nurse leader must translate the philosophy and mission to the staff. It is only through this common viewpoint that leadership and staff, regardless of years of experience and level of education, can come together in a meaningful manner and set common goals and expectations. Without clarity of goals, staff may never understand the expectations of their role or the levels of accountability, productivity, and autonomy to which they are being held.

Most health care organizations' mission statements include some combination of the phrase ". . . provision of cost-effective quality patient care." How is this translated to the staff who is at the point of service and really making a difference in whether patient care is carried out in a cost-effective manner while providing the highest quality of care? How does the staff integrate into their practice the same values that are so dear to the administration?

Nursing administration contributes to the accomplishment of the mission by identifying desired outcomes, providing the most productive and capable personnel within allocated budgets and recommending other nonpersonnel resources that enhance quality in the most cost-effective manner. The staff must then make appropriate decisions in the utilization of supplies and other resources to fulfill the organization's mission and achieve desired outcomes. This means that roles must be clearly defined and outcomes delineated. This is the way that the care providers will recognize the contribution they are making to obtaining desired results. The desired outcomes need to be quality- and cost-specific.

One approach to enable the staff and administration to share the same vision is open communication through the ranks (Champy, 1995). In this way, the staff receives essential information regarding availability of resources, budgetary constraints, and changes that are affecting the way the organization can or cannot operate. It is only with this knowledge that staff can be expected to make the appropriate decisions related to patient care. Information also must be elicited from the staff to assist administration in planning. It is through these open channels of communication that an organization can enhance the effectiveness of its operations.

Another approach to foster the same values among staff and administration is the decentralization of decision-making as appropriate to the nursing role. This forces staff to become accountable because the decision rests in their hands; it is not filtered down to them by a "central office" which the staff may perceive as not having a clue about what is really going on in patient care areas. In order for this approach to be successful, the staff needs information. Goals need to be clear, available resources defined, and the standards of role expectations must be concisely described. Staff must be held to these standards.

Some nurses will be willing to accept the new level of accountability and will develop beyond expectations. Some will develop within the standards and fulfill the expectations. Some will be unwilling or unable to accept the new level of accountability and they will resist additional responsibilities. In a decentralized model, all participants must share equally and those who don't need to be dropped from the organization. A person's inability to value commitment and "ownership" in a job is incompatible with the needs of today's health care organizations which need to move to the next millennium with a work force that shares values and adapts to quick change.

Each nurse, regardless of education and experience, brings a different dimension to the health care setting. With this in mind, new graduates are necessary to assimilate into organizations. With them come fresh ideas and new visions. Nurse leaders must be creative in fostering their growth and development. Some of the newly established nurse intern programs offered by hospitals are excellent vehicles with which to accomplish this task. Experienced nurses need to be held to standards of accountability. Nurses are independent practitioners who must make independent decisions and be accountable for their own practice. The old vision of the "head nurse" being responsible for the practice of all the nurses on a unit is unrealistic in the complexity of today's health care environment. By providing appropriate resources through education, personnel and policies, the nurse leader can enable the staff to perform at this level of independence.

Each nurse needs not only to share the vision of the organization, but also to be a voice in how the mission is operationalized. The nursing leader needs to make this possible by providing the staff with the information and authority to make decisions that are cohesive with the mission. For some leaders this is difficult because the sharing of information and the delegating of certain decision-making is often thought of as a loss of power (Heinbuch & Bedrosian, 1995). On the contrary, the organization is only as strong as every person in it. The degree to which a nursing leader fosters the development of the nursing staff to be independent in practice and make informed and intelligent decisions is the degree to which the staff becomes accomplished in carrying out the mission and vision of the institution.

REFERENCES

Champy, J. (1995). *Reengineering management: The mandate for new leadership.* New York: Harper Business.

Evans, K., Aubrey, K., Hawkins, M., Curley, T., & Porter-O'Grady, T. (1995). Whole systems shared governance: A model for the integrated health system. *Journal of Nursing Administration, 25*(5), 18–27.

Heinbuch, S., & Bedrosian, H. (1995). Reflections on leading the elite. In *Decennial management review of CIOS-World management council.* London: Kensington.

Porter-O'Grady, T. (1994). Building partnerships in health care: Creating whole system change. *Nursing Health Care, 15*(1), 34–38.

The View From Nursing Staff

Cynthia Caroselli

> I can't believe they really want us to change the way we give nurs-
> ing care. How can they possibly know what it's like to work here?
> They *don't* know because they're never on the units—they're
> always in meetings! Nobody knows what a great nurse I really
> am except the people who work side by side with me. I guess
> what I think just doesn't matter around here—why doesn't any-
> one understand what I need?

Sound familiar? Feel familiar? In this turbulent time of health care
upheaval, many nurses spend a considerable part of their professional lives feeling downtrodden, unappreciated, and misunderstood.
Often, individuals experiencing this complex set of emotions will
feel that they are utterly alone, that no one else shares their feelings,
and that those in authority do not understand them. While health
care professionals in various disciplines may share these dispirited
feelings, wallowing in such feelings is depressing, counter-produc-
tive, and self-perpetuating.

TURNING COMPLAINTS INTO NEEDS

John Kenneth Galbraith (1983), noted economist and author, has
said that all great leaders have one characteristic in common, the
ability to respond to the anxieties of their people in their time. This
implies a willingness to hear complaints and to formulate a response
that acknowledges the anxiety as well as provides a resolution of the
problem. From a different perspective, Mick Jagger has noted that
while you can't always get what you want, if you try, you can sometimes get what you need. Neither perspective suggests that one's
needs get addressed through the clairvoyance of the leader. This is
especially true for the professional nurse, regardless of education or

organizational level. Needs and concerns must be communicated to the appropriate person, not merely left to fester and grow.

In the scenario above, the staff member assumes that the administrator is fully aware of the problem and simply chooses to ignore the issue. This assumption may have no basis in reality. Nurses need to be educated to communicate needs in an efficient manner. Students need to become accustomed to helping supervisors (and faculty members, for that matter) understand their needs and to ask questions such as: Is there a knowledge gap that prevents the boss from understanding? Are there resources available to close this knowledge gap? For instance, what published material may help to explain or describe the situation? Sometimes, description is nearly as valuable as a solution in that it gives a name to a phenomenon, acknowledges its existence, and makes communication about the issue more likely. Academic, theoretical material may serve some needs, especially well-constructed studies that allow generalizations from the theoretical to the highly specific; however, anecdotal reports can also prove helpful by describing how others have dealt with similar situations. Students should also become socialized to the value of networking on both macro and micro levels. For instance, large consortium groups, such as the Consortium of Academic Medical Centers, can provide access to large databases of information from similar settings which can assist the individual to formulate solutions. On an individual level, specialty groups can provide a much-needed network for information as well as social support.

THE ROLE OF THE FOLLOWER: NOT THE SAME AS SLUG

While nurses who enter educational programs to prepare for management positions fully expect to exert leadership functions, other graduate nursing students may never consider leadership functions as part of their professional repertoires. This is somewhat surprising, since only approximately 7% of the nation's registered nurses hold master's degrees (U.S. Dept. of Health and Human Services, 1992). Given this number, as well as the curricula and terminal objectives of master's programs, it is clear that master's degree graduates by definition are meant to function as leaders. Yet, many of these individuals do not think of themselves as leaders and are quite emphatic in defining themselves as followers. It is important to recognize, however, that even followership demands a great deal of participation. Followership is most emphatically not a passive role in today's health care environment. Bennis (1994) notes that leaders need direction from followers, which implies that followers need to communicate much information about environmental/organizational issues, clinical issues, and trends, as well as personal needs related to role enactment. This is what Pagonis (1992) terms the interactive nature of leadership and followership.

In essence, this means that all nurses, regardless of relationship to the formal management structure, must travel on the same journey to excellence in patient care. Currently, the nurse practices in an evolving environment. Kerfoot (1996) suggests that, in order to participate in this new world order, one must be a change leader. This role is available to the informal leader as well as those in officially designated management positions. The informal leader may provide a voice for a number of individuals, and may be in possession of unique information or perspectives related to the mission of the organization, which can be invaluable to the formal leader. If every nurse in the organization aspires to informal leadership for at least a portion of his/her professional life, then the collective energy of the group is available for the gargantuan task of meeting patient needs in a time of fiscal constraint. In addition, the scenario that began this discussion is less likely to occur if the reciprocal relationship between leader and follower is enacted. In this way, nurses are less likely to feel as if they are "out of the loop" and thus victimized by management.

This definition of followership relates to the notion of knowledge development as a model for organizational communication. Knowledge development, generally seen as the domain of researchers and theoreticians, can serve as a useful metaphor for organizational communication and relationships. Popper's (1965) groundbreaking work on the growth of scientific knowledge describes a process by which ideas progress from problem to problem. Thus, information develops and deepens as it is explored, and can only be accepted through conjectures and refutations. To operationalize this from an organizational perspective, it can be said that as the nonmanager shares information with the manager, the knowledge is further developed by the manager, who, through reciprocal relationships with non-managers, learns more about the issue or problem, and then digs deeper for more data which either confirm or invalidate the original information. At each successive step, the manager learns more through dialog and fact-finding. Similarly, the nonmanager has the opportunity to influence the manager's knowledge base, participate more fully in the flow of information and activities, and thus influence the work of the organization. This is analogous to what Mintzberg (1996) refers to as craft management which is based on mutual respect and common understanding. Ideally, this taps into the core ideology of the organization, which is what holds an organization together as it grows (Collins & Porros, 1996). If everyone, not just administrators, understands and lives the core values of the organization, then all can more fully participate in the flow of information and direction of core activities.

INTERDISCIPLINARY PERSPECTIVES

Similar to the feeling of being misunderstood by one's administrator is the feeling that other disciplines are antagonistic to nursing and nurses, and are engaged in attempts to eradicate or diminish nursing as we know it. While in some instances this perception may be accurate, it is counterproductive if it becomes the predominant mode of thinking. Most significantly, it perpetuates the "vertical silo" mentality that has been responsible for the demise of many organizations and careers. If nurses persist in this thinking, they will miss opportunities to collaborate in the creation of the "seamless" health care environment.

Being effective in the emerging health care environment means being open to new realities and to understanding, in a practical and concrete way, what these new realities mean for the specific setting in which the nurse practices. New circumstances and new roles present both risks and opportunities. Awareness of both variables allows the creation of solutions. As noted above, solutions can be found in creating new ways in which professionals from various disciplines collaborate to facilitate patient-driven, user-friendly care. Collaboration, however, means more than learning facts about another profession's education or conceptual framework. It means that ". . . we need to understand how others see the world, their motivations, emotions, and aspirations. To see a problem in a new light, we need to analyze it from perspectives other than our own . . . to put ourselves in other people's shoes and to see the world from their point of view" (Fisher, Kopelman, & Schneider, 1994, p. 21). While this has obvious implications for the current flurry of redesign activities, it has broader implications for survival in a time of fiscal constraint.

EDUCATIONAL PERSPECTIVES

Those returning to school to obtain advanced academic credentials need to understand that, while their reasons for wanting an advanced education might be the same as they've always been for nurses, the expectations and eventual outcomes will be radically different. In the past, some nurses may have returned for a graduate degree simply because their employer provided tuition reimbursement benefits. This was also a time when such benefits were provided on a tax-free basis. Current budget constraints and changes in tax laws have resulted in greatly reduced or restricted tuition reimbursement benefits. Some institutions will now reimburse only for those programs that directly relate to the employee's role. This means that potential students need to have a clear idea of their role preparation and its expected outcome *before* they begin. In this way, students can choose programs wisely, and can communicate their needs so that faculty can more specifically structure the educational experience, especially clinical practice.

Regardless of specialty, preparation for a graduate degree should include the development of critical thinking skills, data management skills, and platform skills that allow the graduate to act as an organizational citizen in a new, highly competitive environment. With these skills, the graduate will not only be able to enact role implementation at a high level, but will also be equipped to communicate needs, activities, and information in a way that enables a meaningful response. Articulation of these needs may relate to those of the graduate's constituency or may be related to the nurse's own needs for development.

Similarly, outcomes of graduate nursing programs should include the ability to act as a change master, a collaborator, and an outcomes manager, through a knowledge of cost-effectiveness as it relates to the particular role and function of the area of specialty. While these outcomes may seem purely administrative at first glance, they are essential skills for success in the emerging health care environment. They are particularly relevant when considering the perspective of theorists and practitioners who see a role for all nurses in assuring quality and managing fiscal resources, and no longer see it as the domain of those in traditional management and quality assurance roles.

In light of the above, nursing administration education must include course work related to traditional problem identification, as well as developing expertise in communication that elicits problems and concerns from the constituency. The conceptual approach must center around the notion that administrators and managers must live in the center of the organization, not at the top of it. In this way, communication is facilitated, the opportunity for mutual influence becomes greater, and colleagues become more familiar with each other as individuals, all of which can decrease the alienation sometimes experienced by those in a bureaucratic environment.

Interdisciplinary collaboration and conflict management are critically important skills in the development of a team-based approach to organizational management and redesign. Related to this but perhaps more important is the development of a personal philosophy of what collaboration and the development of mutual respect actually mean in "real life." Most graduate programs in nursing administration as well as other nursing programs have usually included terminal objectives that included ideas similar to "developing a personal philosophy of nursing practice that is grounded in a humanistic approach." New times demand new approaches; however, times of fiscal restraint demand value clarification so that priorities can be thoughtfully established. While some may scoff that such philosophical rumination is "fluff" and that time is better spent honing skills related to such concrete topics as finance, we live in a time of hard choices and difficult decisions. Having to clarify one's values every time one is confronted with an ethical or moral dilemma harkens back to a time before ethics committees and institutional review boards, a time when "reinventing the wheel" was a necessity and there was little on which to rely in terms of concepts, values, or precedents. Time spent by the aspiring administrator considering values and ethics in relation to goals and strategies could actually be an efficient way to prepare for enactment of these activities "for real" at a later time.

CONCLUSION

Those entering the nursing profession today, as well as those reentering it after obtaining new credentials, would do well to see the current health care environment for what it is—radically different from what it was 5 years ago, and evolving through changes that will leave it even more changed 5 years in the future. Nurses who depend on the clairvoyance of their administrators to address needs for development or to enhance clinical practice will find themselves alienated from the organization, or possibly downsized. Those who practice as change leaders, regardless of organizational role, will find their opportunities maximized and their perspectives enlarged. Change will be a factor of professional practice until the end of time—one can deal with it or one can roll over and be acted upon. The choice is open, and the opportunities for vision abound.

REFERENCES

Bennis, W. (1994). *On becoming a leader.* Reading, MA: Addison-Wesley.
Collins, J. C., & Porros, J. I. (1996). Building your company's vision. *Harvard Business Review, 74*(5), 65–77.
Fisher, R., Kopelman, E., & Schneider, A. K. (1994). *Beyond Machiavelli: Tools for coping with conflict.* New York: Penguin Books.
Galbraith, J. K. (1983). *The anatomy of power.* Boston: Houghton Mifflin.
Kerfoot, K. (1996). The new nursing leader for the new world order of health care. *Nursing Economics, 14,* 239–240.
Mintzberg, H. (1996). Musings on management. *Harvard Business Review, 74*(4), 61–67.
Pagonis, W. (1992). The work of the leader. *Harvard Business Review, 70*(6), 118–126.
Popper, K. R. (1965). *Conjectures and refutations: The growth of scientific knowledge.* New York: Harper and Row.
U.S. Dept. of Health and Human Services. (1992). *The registered nurse population: Findings from the national survey of registered nurses 1992.* Washington, DC: U.S. Government Printing Office.

CHAPTER 9

Acute Care Nurse Practitioners: An Idea Whose Time Has Come?

Point

Joan E. King

As with all change, there are pros and cons with health care change. While many struggle with changes in the health care system and the focus on cost containment, these changes have in fact helped to remove the walls and expand the boundaries for advanced practice in nursing. As the fight for health care dollars has progressed, it has become evident that the traditional methods of providing care must change. Patients can no longer remain hospitalized "just to see if they will do well," or because tradition has indicated that patients should remain hospitalized for a predetermined number of days. Hence, traditional approaches to care are being questioned. Perhaps patients really would do well at home in their own environment, provided the patient and family are given enough guidance and education about managing their own care as well as being alert to possible complications. Questioning traditional approaches to care have also included questioning whether certain procedures or skills can be performed by master's degree prepared nurses who have been specially educated, or whether technical skills and procedures must stay under the purview of physicians. Although questioning former practices has added stress

Note: Originally published in *Nursing Leadership Forum*, Vol. 3, No. 3, 1998. New York: Springer Publishing Company.

to the health care system, it has also paved the way for the development of a new advanced practice role: the role of the Acute Care Nurse Practitioner (ACNP).

Historically, nurse practitioners are master's degree prepared nurses who have practiced in primary health care settings focusing on maintenance of health and wellness. Since more patients are being discharged from the hospital sooner, and acute and chronic illnesses are being treated more and more on an outpatient basis, the role for the Acute Care Nurse Practitioner has emerged. It truly is an idea whose time has come.

As stated in the *Standards of Clinical Practice and Scope of Practice for the Acute Care Nurse Practitioner* (American Nurses Association and American Association of Critical Care Nurses, 1995), the purpose of the ACNP is to provide care to patients who are chronically, acutely or critically ill throughout their illness, regardless of setting. This implies that ACNPs practice in a wide variety of settings, including critical care units, emergency departments', acute and subacute units, specialty clinics, and other outpatient settings such as a hospice.

Within these various settings, the ACNP's practice takes on a number of different roles that provide and direct the patient's care and facilitate and accelerate the patient's return to optimal health. First, ACNPs provide direct patient care, not only in terms of traditional nursing care, but also advanced practice care including performing histories and physicals, developing differential diagnoses and problem lists, and developing therapeutic plans of care to meet the patient's needs. Therapeutic plans of care incorporate traditional nursing interventions, such as monitoring vital signs, turning, coughing and deep breathing with advanced practice. For example, therapeutic plans of care also incorporate ordering and interpreting diagnostic and laboratory tests, ordering pharmacological interventions within the guidelines of protocols, and in-depth patient and family teaching. Thus, the therapeutic plans of care blend a holistic nursing focus with the medical model.

The second broad area for practice within the role of the ACNP is to facilitate the coordination of patient care and provide continuity of care by working collaboratively with the physician and other members of the health care team. By rounding with the multidisciplinary team and assessing the patient's progress, the ACNP helps to facilitate optimal delivery of care across a variety of settings. Many times the ACNP will become involved in a patient's care in an out-patient setting, then follow and help coordinate the care through hospitalization, and again back to the outpatient setting. This ability to see patients both in clinics and in the hospital, and to follow patients through the course of their illness, makes the ACNP a key individual for ensuring that the goal of continuity of care is achieved.

The third major component is active participation in the referral process, including identifying the need for consultations and additional services, such as rehabilitation. Since the ACNP's involvement in patient care is not bound by setting, he or she is in an ideal position to identify early in a patient's course of care the need for additional resources and to ensure that these services are incorporated into the patient's care.

The fourth major component of the role of the ACNP encompasses performing very specialized procedures. While all ACNPs may not be involved in settings or patient populations that require utilization of highly technical skills, many ACNPs are. Depending upon where the ACNP practices, he or she may perform specialized procedures, such as harvesting bone marrow, inserting arterial lines, central lines or other access devices, inserting and removing chest tubes, and intubating patients. In the past, these skills have been limited primarily to physicians, but as the health care system has changed, it has become evident that ACNPs are excellent practitioners who can safely and competently perform these skills.

Thus, as the health care system has changed and the complexity of patient care has risen, the door has been opened for the Acute Care Nurse Practitioner. Because of advanced education and a focus on chronic, acute, and critically ill patients, it has become evident that the idea of an Acute Care Nurse Practitioner is one whose time has truly come.

REFERENCE

American Nurses Association and American Association of Critical Care Nurses. (1995). *Standards of clinical practice and scope of practice for the acute care nurse practitioners.* Washington, DC: American Nurses Publishing.

Counterpoint

Barbara J. Daly

The last two decades have been a time of "sea change" in acute care. We have witnessed the shift from retrospective to prospective payment systems, a shift to early discharge and outpatient care, and the overwhelming growth of managed care systems, all stemming from the recognition of an almost panicked response to out-of-control spending. In this unstable environment, all health professions have been engaged in a sometimes desperate effort to keep up, to adapt to the changing demands, and to find effective ways to fulfill our responsibilities to patients in redesigned care systems. Primary nursing came and went, organizational structures were flattened, middle management layers eliminated, and nonlicensed personnel rehired. Our physician colleagues have experienced similar pressures to adapt. Most notably, the inpatient physician work force is threatened by reductions in funding for positions that are primarily education rather than service-oriented, such as specialty fellowships and increasingly stringent requirements for outpatient experiences for residents (Asch & Ende, 1992; Stoddard, Kindig, & Libby, 1994).

Into the breach has come the Acute Care Nurse Practitioner (ACNP). This new role has its origins in two successful traditions: the primary care Nurse Practitioner (NP) and the Clinical Nurse Specialist (CNS). From the inception of the NP role in the early 1960s, under Loretta Ford and Henry Silver at the University of Colorado, research has repeatedly demonstrated the efficiency and effectiveness of this advanced practice role (Brown & Grimes, 1993; Safriet, 1992). The ACNP equally owes its genesis to the CNS role, which demonstrated the effectiveness of having an expert clinician based on hospital units or with specific populations.

The promise and potential of this role is clear. The ACNP represents a solution to the workforce problem. The complement of residents can be reduced or reassigned to outpatient experiences, while the ACNP can provide the constant presence of a knowledgeable clinician at the bedside to manage day-to-day care of patients. This meets the need for close monitoring of patient progress and a partner with whom the busy attending can work. Unlike the medical resident, the ACNP will not be torn by the dual objectives of service and education, will not be constantly rotating to new units, and can be thoroughly integrated as a member of the staff. Perhaps most important, the ACNP will bring his or her nursing perspective to patient management, including an appreciation of the influence of psychosocial factors, the essential need for early and comprehensive discharge planning, and the need to integrate preventive strategies aimed at wellness with curative strategies aimed at disease.

This does, indeed, seem to be an idea whose time has come. But as with most exciting innovations, the devil lies in the detail of application. There are three dangers or misdirections that are very real possibilities. First, because the ACNP does, in fact, substitute or replace resident positions in department budgets, there is a tendency to envision the ACNP role as an almost equivalent substitute for the physician role. If this were true, of course, we could merely subtract residents and add ACNPs, while leaving the system around these roles intact. This would be a great disservice to all involved. It underestimates and underappreciates the depth of education and knowledge gained by physicians in 8–10 years of education and training, which is not equivalent to 5 years of nursing education. Clearly, there is much shared knowledge and overlap in capabilities, particularly between relatively inexperienced physicians and very experienced nurse practitioners. But a nurse is not a physician and acutely ill patients will always have some needs that require physician management. Because of these differences, it is a mistake to expect that ACNPs can be substituted for physicians without any alteration in the complex organizational structure in which they work. A careful evaluation of the need for new policies, new operational routines, and the impact of the role should accompany the introduction of any new role to those with whom the ACNP works.

On the other hand, in some settings the differences between ACNPs and physicians are overestimated. Lack of appreciation of the shortcomings of the current acute care system in comprehensively addressing the health needs of persons, rather than addressing only critical dysfunction of organ systems, is unlikely to promote full utilization of the ACNP's strengths and capabilities. Faced with growing demands on time and shrinking resources, it is understandable that a physician may seek a skilled, knowledgeable assistant to whom s/he can delegate some routine tasks. This is a perfectly understandable need and reasonable solution to a workforce problem. And it should be met by hiring a physician assistant, not an advanced practice nurse.

The third very concerning trend that is accompanying the rapid growth in numbers of ACNPs is a decrease in the use of CNSs. In 1992, ANA reported that there were approximately 40,000 Clinical Nurse Specialists and 30,000 NPs (American Nurses Association, 1992). By 1996, the number of CNSs had increased by 32%, to 53,000, while the number of Nurse practitioners had increased to 63,000, a growth of 110% (Health Professions and Services Administration, 1996). While questions can always be raised about exactly how many CNSs are needed and about productivity of individuals, it seems undeniable that orientation of new staff, providing ongoing education, and evaluating and monitoring standards of nursing care are legitimate and essential functions. One of the strengths of our profession has been our history of preparing professionals for both clinical responsibilities as well as role functions—educator, administrator, consultant. It appears that we are now willing to follow in the footsteps of other professions and either assume that anyone can perform these roles or simply sacrifice these indirect care functions entirely.

These challenges are inevitable but our response to them need not be. The ACNP role is a nursing role, with both limitations and excellence. If we aim to prepare and provide an equivalent physician substitute, we are doomed to failure; our practitioners would always be inadequate. If we are clear, however, about what physician functions an NP cannot assume and what additional improvements in care the ACNP can make, we can build systems that better serve our patients and address some of the demands that are stressing both the acute care organization and other professionals.

Creating new roles and making deep system changes requires the ideas and commitment of more than the nursing department. Planning and initiating a place for ACNPs in the complex bureaucracy of a hospital, with its tripartite mission of service, education, and research, must be a collaborative project. Dropping an ACNP into a structure without adequate consultation from others, such as staff nurses, attending physicians, and house staff coordinators, can be done, but is likely to result in either a nurse in a physician assistant role or a junior house officer.

Being a pioneer can be exciting, but it can also be a lonely, isolating experience. If we want these new practitioners to not only remain in these roles but also flourish as advanced practice nurses, we must build in support structures. Continuing education aimed at their unique needs, opportunities to meet and discuss common problems with other advanced practice nurses, guidance, support, and leadership from nursing as well as physician mentors will not happen without specific plans and structures in place.

As a profession, we have much work yet to do. The rationale for the ACNP role is quite clear. The profession has shown an impressive ability to respond to the demands of the marketplace by starting more than 50 ACNP programs in schools of nursing in just the past 5 years, as well as writing a Scope of Practice statement and establishing a certification examination in this specialty. We must now tackle the challenge of evaluating these new graduate programs and the role itself. We have thus far assumed that minor modifications in primary care nurse practitioner programs would adequately prepare graduates for practice in acute care settings, but this has yet to be tested. Continued growth in the numbers of ACNPs is unlikely to occur and should not be encouraged without outcome research demonstrating that this role is contributing to improvements in patient care.

The ACNP role does hold great promise, but it is accompanied by a critical proviso. If we are not up to the task of changing the way care is delivered, using the different perspective, skills, and knowledge base of all advanced practice nurses, then we would be wise not to squander our nursing resources by sacrificing our most skilled practitioners to this limited and narrow role of enabling the status quo.

REFERENCES

American Nurses Association. (1992). *Nursing facts.* Washington, DC: Author.

Asch, D. A., & Ende, J. (1992). The downsizing of internal medicine residency. *Annals of Internal Medicine, 117,* 839–844.

Brown, S. A., & Grimes, D.E. (1993). *A meta-analysis of process of care, clinical outcomes and cost-effectiveness of nurses in primary care roles:*

Nurse practitioners and nurse midwives. Prepared for the ANA Division of Health Policy. Washington, DC: American Nurses Association.

Health Professions and Services Administration. (1996, March). HHS BHPr advance notes from the national sample of registered nurses [On-line]. Available: http://www.hrsa.dhhs.gov/bhpr/dn/advnote1. htm

Safriet, B. (1992). Health care dollars and regulatory sense: The role of advanced practice nursing. *Yale Journal of Regulation, 9,* 417–488.

Stoddard, J. J., Kindig, D. A., & Libby, D. (1994). Graduate medical education reform. *Journal of the American Medical Association, 272,* 53–58.

CHAPTER 10

Primary and Secondary Prevention: How Much a Part of Nursing?

Point: Are Nurses Making a Substantial Contribution?

Nancy T. Artinian

Nurses have been making a substantial contribution to primary and secondary prevention since the days of Florence Nightingale. Primary prevention interventions include health promotion and aim to prevent the onset of disease (Rubenstein & Nahas, 1998). Secondary prevention interventions emphasize early diagnosis and prompt treatment and aim to identify an established disease in the presymptomatic stage to cure it early or prevent its progression (Rubenstein & Nahas, 1998). Nursing's contributions to preventive care are evident at all levels and aspects of the profession including leadership and policy development, theory development, practice, and research and scholarship.

Nursing leaders are spearheading initiatives and policies and disseminating knowledge about theories and skills that nurses need to understand when providing care. In 1994 the Office of Disease Prevention and Health Promotion of the Public Health Service of the United States Department of Health and Human Services

Note: Originally published in *Nursing Leadership Forum*, Vol. 5, No. 1, 2000. New York: Springer Publishing Company.

launched a national campaign entitled "Put Prevention into Practice" (United States Public Service [USPHS], 1994). Its mission is to achieve the Healthy People 2000 goal (now Healthy People 2010) of getting clinical preventive services to all Americans. Members of the American Nurses Association, American Association of Colleges of Nursing, and the National Alliance of Nurse Practitioners were actively involved in the development of this national effort and remain actively involved in its implementation (USPHS, 1994).

Nursing leaders helped develop recommendations for cardiac risk factor modification. The Clinical Practice Guidelines for Cardiac Rehabilitation were developed by a private-sector panel convened by the Agency for Health Care Policy and Research (AHCPR, now the Agency for Healthcare Research and Quality) and the National Heart, Lung, and Blood Institute (NHLBI) (1995). Nurses participated in this multidisciplinary panel that was cochaired by Erika Sivarajan Froelicher, RN, PhD. Other nurse leaders concerned about cardiovascular risk reduction organized the Lipid Nurse Task Force, a national multidisciplinary effort to provide professional development, community education, and comprehensive patient care to the millions of Americans who have elevations in total cholesterol (http://www.Intf.org).

Nurse scholars write a voluminous amount about health promotion and disease prevention. From a CINAHL search of the literature from 1982 to 2000, using the keywords "nursing and preventive health care," emerged 25,237 citations. Prominent books in the field include "Health Promotion throughout the Lifespan" (Edelman & Mandle, 1998), "Nurses and Family Health Promotion: Concepts, Assessment and Interventions" (Bomar, 1995), and "Health Promotion in Nursing Practice" (Pender, 1996). Pender's (1996) Health Promotion Model has been used worldwide to guide practice and research.

Nurse clinicians and researchers use individual-level and community-level preventive care interventions with infants, children, adolescents, adults, and elders. A critical role for public health nurses (PHNs) is the surveillance and monitoring of disease trends (Zahner, 1999). One surveillance system in the United States is the National Immunization Survey, a system that methodically collects, analyzes, and interprets child immunization data. PHNs play a key role in this system since they provide and document immunizations as well as use the data from surveillance systems to plan and evaluate immunization programs (Zahner, 1999). Nurses play an important role in supporting local programs to immunize infants and young children through the health teaching they provide to new mothers at delivery and in the interactions that they have for periodic and episodic health care for children (Bellig, 1995). PHNs provide immunizations to nearly half of American children and work to devise creative approaches, such as designing alternative clinics, to take immunization services to more people (Horner & Murphy, 1999). Nurse researchers are concerned with promoting infant and child health and have investigated phenomenon such as prenatal and infancy home visitation services by nurses as a way of improving maternal and child outcomes. Kitzman and colleagues (1997) found that home visitation reduced pregnancy-induced hypertension, childhood injuries, and subsequent pregnancies among low-income women with no previous live births.

Nurses provide preventive care to children and adolescents in other important ways. A few examples include screening and testing for elevated blood lead levels, implementing bicycle safety workshops to raise public awareness about child safety, and providing AIDS and substance use prevention programs (Fisher & Vessey, 1998; Hart & Daughtridge, 1998; Jemmott, 1993; Werch, Pappas, Carlson, & DiClemente, 1999). Nurses are working across a variety of well-child care settings such as schools and clinics assessing cardiovascular health and teaching children and adolescents and their families about ways to prevent cardiovascular disease through healthy eating, not smoking, and engaging in family fitness activities (Hayman & Ryan, 1994). Harrell and associates (1999) conducted a randomized controlled field trial to determine the population effects of both classroom-based and risk-based interventions to reduce cardiovascular risk factors in children. The investigators found that both classroom-based and risk-based interventions had positive effects on physical activity and knowledge.

Nurses provide preventive care to adults and elders in numerous venues. Oncology nurses provide education and counseling about tobacco cessation, reducing sun exposure, diet and weight control, awareness of occupational exposure to carcinogens, recognition of old age as a risk factor, and genetic risk assessment if there is a pattern of familial cancer (Spencer-Cisek, 1998; Varricchio, 1997). Teaching self-detection practices is an important part of what a nurse does to encourage the early detection of cancers. Adult nurse practitioners and women's health nurse practitioners assess for risk factors, conduct screening tests, and implement educational interventions for the prevention of osteoporosis, hypertension, cardiovascular disease, stroke, syndrome X, obesity, diabetes mellitus, and cancer (Masten & Gary, 1999). Several nurse investigators have developed programs of research focused on health promotion and risk reduction in adults (Champion, 1999; Moore, Ruland, Pachkow, & Blackburn, 1998; Nies, Vollman, & Cook, 1998; Rice et al., 1994).

Two thirds of accidents of people older than 65 years are due to falls (Lange, Hintermeister, Schlegal, Dilman, & Steadman, 1996). Gerontological nurses work to identify elderly at risk for falls, encourage physical and social activity and physical fitness, modify the elder's environment, and educate the elders about accident prevention. Promotion of bone health and prevention of osteoporosis is crucial to the prevention of fractures; nurses in various settings provide education and counseling to achieve this aim (Lappe, 1998).

Family violence is another health risk that is a focus of assessment by adult health nurses as well as public health nurses. Nurses work in battered women's shelters providing counseling and parenting education, are involved in school-based violence prevention, and are part of education teams in emergency departments in assessment of family violence (Bekemeier, 1995). Parenting education, modeling of appropriate interactions, and providing direct reassurance for the child are public health nursing interventions that are employed to reduce the negative outcomes of family violence for the child (Bekemeier, 1995).

Occupational health nurses (OHN) work to recognize and evaluate potential and existing health hazards in the workplace, eliminate or minimize workplace hazards, advise employers about health and safety matters, and teach employees how to protect themselves from actual and potential hazards (Lessure & Griffith, 1995). Lusk and colleagues' (1999) research exemplifies the work of occupational health nurses. Over 30 million workers are exposed to hazardous noise on the worksite. Continual exposure to high noise levels damages and destroys hearing cells within the ear. Lusk and associates (1999) have tested the effectiveness of theory-based interventions (video, pamphlets, and guided practice session) to increase the use of hearing protection devices (HPDs) among midwestern construction workers and a national group of plumber/pipefitter trainers.

As the preceding examples show, nurses collectively make a substantial contribution to primary and secondary prevention. Research has documented that nursing's preventive care efforts are successful. Nursing's challenge is to continue to strive to maintain and expand its successes.

REFERENCES

Agency for Health Care Policy and Research and National Heart, Lung, and Blood Institute. (1995). *Clinical practice guideline: Cardiac rehabilitation.* (AHCPR Publication No. 96-0672).

Bekemeier, B. (1995). Public health nurses and the prevention of and intervention in family violence. *Public Health Nursing, 12*(4), 222–227.

Bellig, L. L. (1995). Immunization and the prevention of childhood diseases. *Journal of Obstetrics, Gynecologic, Neonatal Nursing, 24*(7), 669–677.

Bomar, P. J. (1995). *Nurses and family health promotion: Concepts, assessment and intervention* (2nd ed.). Philadelphia: W. B. Saunders.

Champion, V. L. (1999). Revised susceptibility, benefits, and barriers scale for mammography screening. *Research in Nursing and Health, 22*(4), 341–348.

Edelman, C. L., & Mandle, C. L. (1998). *Health promotion throughout the lifespan* (4th ed.). St. Louis: Mosby.

Fisher, A. M., & Vessey, J. A. (1998). Preventing lead poisoning and its consequences. *Pediatric Nursing, 24*(4), 348–350.

Harrell, J. S., McMurray, R. G., Gansky, S. A., Bangdiwala, S. I., & Bradley, C. B. (1999). A public health versus a risk-based intervention to improve cardiovascular health in elementary school children: The Cardiovascular Health in Children Study. *American Journal of Public Health, 89*(10), 1529–1535.

Hart, K. M., & Daughtridge, J. (1998). Implementing a bicycle safety workshop. *Orthopaedic Nursing, 17*(3), 49–52.

Hayman, L. L., & Ryan, E. A. (1994). The cardiovascular health profile: Implications for health promotion and disease prevention. *Pediatric Nursing, 20*(5), 509–516.

Horner, S. D., & Murphy, L. (1999). Creating alternative immunization clinics to maintain and improve community immunization rates. *Journal of Community Health Nursing, 16*(2), 121–132.

Jemmott, L. S. (1993). AIDS risk among black male adolescents: Implications for nursing interventions. *Journal of Pediatric Health Care, 7*(1), 3–11.

Kitzman, H., Olds, D. L., Henderson, C. R., Hanks, C., Cole, R., Tatelbaum, R., McConnochie, K. M., Sidora, K., Luckey, D. W., Shaver, D., Engelhardt, K., James, D., & Barnard, K. (1997). Effect of prenatal and infancy home visitation by nurses on pregnancy outcomes, childhood injuries, and repeated childbearing. *Journal of the American Medical Association, 278*(8), 644–652.

Lange, G. W., Hintermeister, R. A., Schlegal, T., Dilman, C. J., & Steadman, J. R. (1996). Electromyographic and Kinematic analysis of graded treadmill walking and the implications for knee rehabilitation. *Journal of Orthopaedic and Sports Physical Therapy, 23*(5), 294–301.

Lappe, J. M. (1998). Prevention of hip fractures: A nursing imperative. *Orthopaedic Nursing, 17*(3), 15–24.

Lessure, L. J., & Griffith, H. M. (1995). Putting prevention into clinical practice. *American Association of Occupational Health Nurses Journal, 43*(2), 72–75.

Lusk, S. L., Hong, O. S., Ronis, D. L., Eakin, B. L., Kerr, M. J., & Early, M. R. (1999). Effectiveness of an intervention to increase construction workers' use of hearing protection. *Human Factors, 41*(3), 487–494.

Masten, Y., & Gary, A. (1999). Is anyone listening? Does anyone care? Menopausal and postmenopausal health risks, outcomes and care. *Nurse Practitioner Forum, 10*(4), 195–200.

Moore, S. M., Ruland, C. M., Pashkow, F. J., & Blackburn, G. G. (1998). Women's patterns of exercise following cardiac rehabilitation. *Nursing Research, 47*(6), 318–324.

Nies, M. A., Vollman, M., & Cook, T. (1998). Facilitators, barriers, and strategies for exercise in European American women in the community. *Public Health Nursing, 15*(4), 263–272.

Pender, N. J. (1996). *Health promotion in nursing practice* (3rd ed.). Stamford, CT: Appleton & Lange.

Rice, V. H., Fox, D. H., Lepczyk, M., Sieggreen, M., Mullin, M., Jarosz, & Templin, T. (1994). A comparison of nursing interventions for smoking cessation in adults with cardiovascular health problems. *Heart & Lung, 23*(6), 473–486.

Rubenstein, L. Z., & Nahas, R. (1998). Primary and secondary prevention strategies in the older adult. *Geriatric Nursing, 19*(1), 11–18.

Spencer-Cisek, P. A. (1998). Overview of cancer prevention, screening, and detection. *Nurse Practitioner Forum, 9*(3), 134–146.

United States Public Health Service (USPHS). (1994). *Put prevention into action kit.* Washington, DC: Government Printing Office, 017-001-00492-8.

Varricchio, C. G. (1997). Cancer in adults: A focus on prevention and detection in the nurse practitioner's practice. *Nurse Practitioner Forum, 8*(2), 64–69.

Werch, C. E., Pappas, D. M., Carlson, J. M., & DiClemente, C. C. (1999). Six-month outcomes of an alcohol prevention program for inner-city youth. *American Journal of Health Promotion, 13*(4), 237–240.

Zahner, S. J. (1999). Public health nursing and immunization surveillance. *Public Health Nursing, 16*(6), 384–389.

Counterpoint: Isn't Primary Health Care Synonymous With Nursing Practice?

Kimberly Adams-Davis

In 1978, some 134 countries endorsed primary health care as the method for providing acceptable, accessible, and effective health care for the world's peoples. These countries overwhelmingly espoused their belief in the five principles of primary health care including, promotive, preventive (primary, secondary, and tertiary), curative, supportive, and rehabilitative aspects of care. MacIntosh and McCormack assert that:

> Despite this overwhelming endorsement very few countries have made changes in policies and infrastructure for implementing the underlying values and beliefs ascribed in primary health care . . . This delay has resulted in and will continue to have, a huge impact on nursing education, practice, and research. (2000, p. 116)

Mary Breckenridge's Frontier Nursing Service, Lillian Wald's Hale House, Loretta Ford's Pediatric Nurse Practitioner Programs, and many others like them constitute a public health nursing legacy that was founded on principles of primary health care (Komnenich, 1997). Despite this legacy, nursing has not continued to focus on the provision of primary health care. One only has to review the components of primary health care as set forth by the World Health Organization (WHO) to see how far nursing has veered from this legacy. This review of the WHO standards reveals that the essential components of primary care include: (a) health care that reflects and evolves from economic conditions and sociocultural/political characteristics of a community and is based on an appropriate application of social, health care research, and public health experience; (b) health promotion, preventive, curative, and rehabilitative services to address the major health problems of a community; and (c) education specific to the community served, concerning the prevailing health problems and methods to prevent and control them (WHO, 2000).

An assessment of current nursing practice reveals a paucity of primary health care services. Multiple factors contribute to the lack of integration of primary health care concepts in nursing practice. Major factors that impede this integration include (a) educational curricula that center on treatment of disease and that emphasize an acute care focus, (b) a health care system that focuses on acute care, and (c) a reimbursement system that severely restricts reimbursement for health promotion and disease prevention activities. Other factors include staffing patterns in hospitals, clinics, and private offices, as well as the limited primary health care content in current professional nursing journals. These factors will be discussed in the following paragraphs.

The stated philosophies of many schools of nursing espouse a belief in health promotion and disease prevention ". . . to assist individuals to attain, maintain, and regain optimal health" (Glazer & Presslar, 1989), however, often these philosophies are in conflict with the actual curricular content. A review of diploma, AD, BSN, and advanced practice nursing curricula reveals very little subject matter devoted to primary health care concepts such as primary and secondary prevention (immunizations, screening, etc). Nearly three-fourths of the schools of nursing's basic educational curricula center on the diagnosis and treatment of disease, pathophysiology of rare and complex diseases, and administration of medications. Even when academic courses are given titles such as "Well Woman Health Care," "Children and Adolescents in Health & Illness," or "Family Health Nursing: Health of Adults and Older Adults," an examination of course descriptions and reading assignments highlights the acute care focus of these courses. Many nursing schools provide a solely acute care focus during the last year of study. Very little course work emphasizes public, population-focused, and primary health care concepts, such as primary and secondary prevention, health teaching, lifestyle and behavior modification, risk assessment, and community advocacy. These curricular patterns indicate the emphasis on the acute care focus of nursing. This acute care focus continues once the graduate nurse begins to practice.

Although the focus of the United States (U.S.) health care system has shifted from long stays in acute settings to home- and community-based health care, there continues to be a focus on acute care procedures and medical technology. Very little has changed over the past 20 years regarding the U.S. health system policies and infrastructure changes necessary for implementing the foundational beliefs and values underscored in the primary health care principles (MacIntosh & McCormack, 2000). Thus, the majority of nurses continue to practice in acute care settings and focus almost solely on curative and palliative measures. Day-to-day work consists of coordinating diagnostic tests, scheduling therapies, performing treatments, and administering medications. Several workplace challenges exist, such as high patient acuity, reimbursement patterns that favor technology and acute care services rather than prevention, and staffing patterns that result in high nurse-to-patient ratios. These challenges lead to little time for preventative counseling, education regarding disease processes, risk assessment, and the administration of immunizations. In ambulatory settings, once again, high advanced practice nurse to patient ratios, productivity expectations, and reimbursement patterns result in a focus on the management of acute episodes. Attention to primary health care concepts lag far behind. There is little time allotted for the provision of primary care services in the typical 45-minute new visit and the 15-minute episodic or return visit. One example is the nurse midwife who is scheduled to see a total of 25–30 patients per day. This schedule includes women with various management and treatment needs such as pregnancy-induced hypertension, condyloma acuminata, dysfunctional uterine bleeding, and osteoporosis. This leads to little time for educational counseling, screening, and/or anticipatory guidance. This reality results in a focus on acute care issues in practice that also is translated to education settings.

An appraisal of the nursing literature over the past 4 years highlights the acute care focus in the professional literature. A medline search of "primary health care and nursing" produced some 259 journal articles with primary care or primary health care in the title. A review of the journal abstracts often indicated a lack of primary health care content, despite the titles. Most of the authors equated primary health care with ambulatory settings or "first contact" health care providers rather than with the types of service provided. Content subjects such as pharmocokinetics/pharmocodynamics, treatment of disease, and pathophysiology dominated the practice and research literature.

Nurses will only begin to practice primary health care in the fullest sense if educational programs prepare them adequately for careers in primary health care and the health care system infrastructure and values are revised to support the provision of primary health care. Lastly, nursing leaders have to advocate for and support the practice of primary health care through shaping of the content of nursing curricula, leading the movement to provide evidence-based research focusing on primary health care, and creating a critical mass of literature that focuses on primary health care concepts, principles, and practice exemplars.

REFERENCES

Glazer, G., & Presslar, J. (1989). Schlotfeldt's health seeking nursing model. In J. Fitzpatrick and A. Whall (Eds.), *Conceptual models of nursing* (pp. 241–253). Norwalk, CT: Appleton & Lange.

Komnenich, P. (1997). The evolution of advanced practice in nursing. In C. M. Sheehy and M. C. McCarthy (Eds.). *Advanced practice nursing: Emphasizing common roles* (pp. 8–46). Philadelphia: F. A. Davis.

MacIntosh, J., & McCormack, D. (2000). An integrative review illuminates curricular applications of primary health care. *Journal of Nursing Education, 39*(3), 116–123.

World Health Organization. (2000, June 3) *International Conference in Alma-Ata, USSR* [On-line]. Available: http://www.who. int/aboutwho/en/history.htm

CHAPTER 11

Unlicensed Personnel: A Threat to Nursing and Patients?

Point: Safe in the Right Hands

Darlene L. Cox

Nursing has used unlicensed personnel throughout its history. Yet today, one hears a cry against this practice.

Change is always threatening, and nursing—as well as the rest of health care—has faced a whirlwind of change in the last decade or two. One of those changes has been the advancement of nursing as a profession as recognized in a very concrete form: greatly increased wages for the nurse at the bedside. No change is without repercussions, and nurses should have anticipated the changes that would be forced on the system by improved salaries. Two facts can't be ignored: (a) nurses constitute the largest class of employees in the majority of health care institutions, and (b) monies coming into health care have not merely remained constant but have been shrunk by systematic manipulation of the system. Put these two facts together and the prediction is easy: If each nurse is to receive more remuneration from a system with shrinking resources, then there will be fewer nurses. That is exactly what has happened, and nurses are crying, "unfair." Yet it is naive to assume that society will turn back the clock

Note: Originally published in *Nursing Leadership Forum*, Vol. 1, No. 2, 1995. New York: Springer Publishing Company.

or put more money into health care simply because nurses don't want to pay the price of their victory.

Simply put, the price of higher salaries is higher expectations of performance. Part of those expectations include more management functions. To be worth more money, the nurse must extend and expand the services she renders, and there's no other way to do it except for managing others. Indeed, the recent ruling that all RNs are managers (under the National Labor Relations Act) is a legal recognition of that change.

Whether nurses like it or not, this society has drawn a line on how much of its resources it wants to spend on providing health care. That decision doesn't reflect the level of care nurses would prefer, all things being equal. But all things aren't equal. Society has given us a clear mandate: Do the best you can with what you receive.

Doing the best we can means we must cast off the prejudices of the past and think care delivery anew. The traditional nurse's aide position has, for the most part, outlived its usefulness in today's high-tech environment. Yet there is no reason that assistive personnel cannot extend the services of each nurse if—and this is the important one—they are fully trained to do the things they are required to do, and if they are adequately supervised.

No one is saying that unlicensed personnel can replace nurses; no one is saying that they should work unsupervised. To argue that they *do* work unsupervised is to fault the system, not the principle.

Nurses get scared when today's technician is taught more complex tasks than yesterday's nurse's aide. Yet ironically, that doesn't mean the tech is less safe, less prepared. Technology has created many new tasks that may appear more difficult than the old nurse's aide passing out lunch trays. Yet the levels of difficulty may not be what they seem. Indeed, the old task of passing out lunch trays demanded more knowledge (who should have salt on what diet, who shouldn't be eating because a test requiring NPO was ordered). In comparison, a technically complex procedure, done over and over again—like irrigating a feeding tube—has fewer decision points and is certainly less complex than driving a car—a skill this society admits an 18-year old can learn.

The American Association of Critical Care Nurses (AACN; 1990) has given us a perfectly good set of criteria for judging when a technician may safely perform a task. The criteria are:

1. The potential for harm
2. The complexity of the nursing activity
3. The required problem-solving and innovation
4. The predictability of outcome
5. The extent of patient interaction

The issue is not whether the criteria make sense—they do. The issue is whether they are applied accurately. When an institution fails in the application, it makes no sense to indict the criteria.

Nursing management has been faced with tremendous demands in this era of constricting resources. Sometimes we are strained to find the way. We are aware of the stress nurses face when asked to do more and more. We are also aware that they can only be stretched so far. Nursing had to find an answer, and we did: restructured practice. Restructured practice, although it is a response to a tough situation, has been healthy for the profession because it has forced us to set aside our earlier assumptions and look at the whole process of delivering care anew and fresh.

In setting aside old assumptions, we recognized a truth about modern managing: that the profession had become a de facto series of subprofessions, namely specialties. It is no longer true that a nurse is a nurse is a nurse—if it ever were true. Today, every vice president for nursing knows that she cannot send a nurse who specializes in endocrinology to an orthopedic unit. If she does, the expectations are not that the nurse will be fully functional. This is the price of today's specialism.

Yet restructured practice allows us to extend the fact of specialism down the line to the categories of assistive personnel. Instead of one generalized nurse's aide, we have various technicians, taught the skills of a specialized practice, able to do more technologically complex skills (skills selected on AACN criteria, for example), for a more narrow range of patients.

Some object to assistive personnel because there are no standard guidelines for what they may do. To standardize their tasks would prevent the use of them as specialist aides. The standards are in the criteria, not in the tasks.

No one is saying that restructured practice, with its heavy use of assistive personnel, gives us a perfect world. But the fact of the matter is that we aren't asked to give care in a perfect world. We are asked to give care in a resource-scarce world, and we are asked to do the best we can with it.

The best we can do is offer effective use of assistive personnel. For others to say that this is unprofessional begs the question. The question is not, "What is ideal nursing?" but, "What is the best way to get the most out of our shrinking resources?"

Arguments against use of assistive personnel are miscast when we hear that these assistants were employed to free nurses to plan and evaluate. That has the cart before the horse. When assistive personnel must be used (like today), then one asks, "What are the most critical tasks of nursing?" and "What tasks must be kept for the professional?" Planning and evaluation can't be done by lower levels, mechanical tasks can—even if they constitute much of "hands-on" nursing.

One of the problems in the transition to use of subordinate personnel is that nurses are not yet being prepared for the new role they will assume. They must be taught how to work with subordinates, how to oversee their work, safeguard their patients, and, among other skills, learn how to delegate and exercise authority with comfort.

One fear is that the "hospital" is taking over, deciding what assistive personnel can and can't do. Yet in every case, it is the nursing department that decides on the assistive tasks. The hospital, or its administration, can hardly be held up as the enemy. Indeed, nursing proved itself very strong when someone else, namely, medicine, tried to take over its turf in the form of the registered care technician proposal.

Nursing won the battle to manage nursing; nursing won the high salaries. If nursing wants more resources put into health care so that more nursing personnel may be employed, this issue—like others—must be taken to the public at large.

Some claim that the problem could be solved by simply allotting tasks differently among nurses according to their education preparation rather than by using auxilliary personnel. This begs the question. Divide RNs any way you want, and they still cost too much (given our resources). Yes, a hospital can increase its nursing budget—but it can also go belly-up when its costs are higher than any insurance company deigns to pay.

The "stand pats" among our nurse peers fail to see the world we live in is changing. They fault use of assistive personnel because some use these personnel wrongly. Some fail at marriage too—should we eliminate it? Or motherhood? Or teaching? Should assistive personnel function without proper supervision? No, of course not. Should the nurse earning $40,000 or $50,000 per annum expect to have to supervise others? Yes. Should she learn how to do it properly? By all means. Should the nursing management of every institution control the practice of subordinate nurse technician staff, including determining what tasks these nonprofessionals can and cannot do? Yes. Assistive personnel may not be the ideal solution in patient care, but they are a feasible solution in today's very difficult situation.

REFERENCE

American Association of Critical Care Nurses. (1990). *Delegation of nursing and nonnursing activities in critical care.* Alison Viejo, CA: Author.

Counterpoint: Unlicensed to Care

Mary Jane Kalafut DiMattio

> The untrained nurse is as old as the human race; the trained
> nurse is a recent discovery. The distinction between the two is
> a sharp commentary on the follies and prejudices of mankind.
> (Robinson in Donohue, 1985, p. 1)

It is disturbing to realize that the above passage, published in 1946, has new meaning in 1995 as the proliferation and misuse of unlicensed assistive personnel in hospitals threaten the status of professional nursing. The use of unlicensed personnel poses an insidious threat to nursing, and it would be wise for the profession to fight to preclude these personnel from providing direct patient care.

In theory, unlicensed assistive personnel support the registered nurse in the delivery of nursing care. They provide both indirect care, such as stocking supplies, and direct care, such as feeding and bathing patients (American Nurses' Association [ANA], 1993). There are, however, no standard guidelines for hiring or training these individuals, and some hospitals plan to incorporate "multiskilled caregivers" who would assist RNs by performing activities ranging from vital signs to simple dressing changes ("Layoffs loom," 1994). The rationale for the use of assistive personnel is to free registered nurses to plan and evaluate patient care, resulting in more efficient and cost-effective hospital stays (ANA, 1993; Barter & Furmidge, 1994). The reality, however, is that cost savings due to increased use of assistive personnel is not a well established fact (Manuel & Alster, 1994). In one study, only 1 hospital of the 67 surveyed reported "multiple measures" of the cost-effectiveness of assistive personnel (Barter, McLaughlin, & Thomas, 1994).

Registered nurses are accountable for delegating all activities to unlicensed personnel (ANA, 1993; Barter & Furmidge, 1994). The ANA (1993) defines delegation as "the transfer of responsibility for the performance of an activity from one person to another while retaining accountability for the outcome" (p. 2). The ANA (1993) also states that the nursing profession defines the utilization of unlicensed assistants for patient care. Historically, however, hospital hierarchies have benefited from a tradition of domination and control over nursing (Roberts, 1983). Staff nurses are still fighting for autonomy in hospitals and are generally not included in policy decisions (Schmieding, 1993). It is therefore unrealistic to think that nurses are being asked to formulate job descriptions for unlicensed personnel. Schmieding (1993) stated that delegation empowers nurses as long as it takes place in the context of authority and autonomy in practice, but the use of unlicensed assistants by hospitals for direct patient care does damage to the concept of delegation and squelches nurse empowerment. When hospitals confer responsibilities upon assistive personnel, knowing that nursing is legally accountable for the activities of these individuals, nurses are forced into a situation of responsibility without authority. Registered nurses have no say as to the utilization of assistive personnel but shoulder the blame when untoward circumstances occur.

The use of unlicensed personnel is deeply intertwined with another major threat to nursing's power and autonomy. Recently, the Supreme Court ruled that nurses who supervise individuals of lesser skill are considered managers and are not afforded the right to organize and bargain under the National Labor Relations Act (NLRA). In addition, nurses will no longer be protected under the NLRA in disputing labor practices in hospitals. Under this ruling, individual hospitals will undoubtedly take every opportunity to prevent nurses from organizing against unfair working conditions ("Striking at bargaining rights," 1994), including refusal to supervise unlicensed personnel.

The use of unlicensed personnel in situations of inadequate staffing by RNs also erodes nursing's power base. Inadequate staffing, a situation plaguing many hospitals, makes true delegation a myth even among licensed nurses. Adding unskilled personnel presents the real threat that these individuals will not be adequately supervised, and that their activities will exceed their preparation. The ANA (1993) expressed concern over assistive personnel performing tasks that legally fall into the scope of nursing practice "in virtually all health care settings" (p.1). Ultimately, nursing loses control over quality of care, and patients are endangered.

Quality care is of paramount importance when examining the issue of unlicensed personnel because it is toward this end that all of nursing scholarship is dedicated. By hiring unlicensed individuals to provide patient care, hospitals send the message that there is little difference between the professional and the nonprofessional outside of what is delineated by law. This accomplishes much in the way of illustrating that attitudes toward organized nursing have not changed much in over 100 years.

Because nursing has traditionally been associated with the female role, and because the activities that constitute the art and science of nursing are deeply contextual (Benner, 1984), nursing has struggled to prove the need for its members to be well-educated. Florence Nightingale's idea for a training school for nurses at the St. Thomas Hospital in London was met with opposition from many in high society, including medical professionals. To the latter group, nurse training in the hands of nurses was an affront because physicians controlled the so-called training of nurses at the time (Nutting & Dock, 1907, vol. 2, chap. 3). Furthermore, the need for well-trained nurses was not deemed necessary. "As regards the nurses or wardmaids, these are in much the same position as housemaids and require little teaching" (Nutting & Dock, 1907, vol. 2, p. 181). Nurse training faced some of the same difficulties in America as it did in Europe. For example, the training school at the Massachusetts General Hospital was initially unwanted by the medical staff and considered to be too disruptive to the running of the wards. Were it not for the strong leadership of Linda Richards, the school would probably not have survived (Nutting & Dock, 1907, vol. 2, chap. 8).

A century later, hospital hierarchies are still challenging the need for educated nurses in the name of monetary savings, while other costs to patients are not even being considered. The nursing function that stands to be most endangered by unlicensed personnel providing direct care to patients is what Benner (1984) called the "diagnostic and monitoring function." This function is vital to the well-being of patients and is central to the nurse's role because the nurse spends the most time with patients (Benner, 1984, chap. 6). Nurses are in the best position to recognize progress as well as deterioration and to forestall complications. Time studies and efficiency experts cannot measure how much a nurse can determine about a patient's welfare during brief encounters for seemingly simple activities because a nurse's judgment represents a hybrid of experience informed by a scientific knowledge base (Benner, 1984). The more time the nurse spends away from the patient, the greater the likelihood that subtle cues to changes in that patient's condition will be missed. A recent case in point occurred in a California hospital when a patient suffered insulin shock due to the failure of an unlicensed individual to recognize the symptoms ("Gallup finds," 1994).

Many argue that nurses cannot possibly do everything for their patients. This is true when "everything" includes running to the pharmacy for missing medications, filling water pitchers, and transporting patients. This is also true when there is no housekeeping staff on the weekends to clean rooms and empty trash. Also, when nurses spend an inordinate amount of time providing what Schmieding (1993) termed "physician monitoring service," there is less time to spend with patients. Schmieding (1993) pointed out that physicians do not have to remind nurses to do parts of their jobs! It simply defies common sense that professional nurses are still performing all of the above tasks while hospitals bring in unlicensed individuals to care for the patients. There is no reason to prevent unlicensed personnel from performing indirect care activities, but as a profession, nursing is being denied the right to provide high-quality care informed by nursing theory, research, and experience. Would a law firm suggest that its lawyers assign legal aides to try "minor" cases, or would an airline allow flight attendants to fly planes in good weather? Never! But making such seemingly ridiculous comparisons serves to illustrate the point that nurses still need to fight for treatment as professionals in hospital settings.

Undoubtedly, hospital and health care costs must be controlled, but reducing the numbers of professional nurses is not the answer. Nurses can find ways to streamline care within their own ranks by using the tiered system of nursing education as it was originally intended (Manuel & Alster, 1994). A movement toward assigning nurses to activities according to the focus of their preparation would utilize nurses' skills appropriately while ensuring that all patients are cared for by properly educated, professional nurses. The emphasis upon the difference in nursing roles according to preparation should begin in educational programs and be reflected in nurse licensing exams.

Perhaps one of nursing's greatest allies in protecting its professionalism is the public that it exists to serve. Roberts (1983) suggested that nurses, as an oppressed group, have experienced difficulty maintaining solidarity and have assimilated with the dominant medical culture in hospitals. Thus, the profession's ideals have not been championed by its members. It is time for nurses to tell the public, starting with family and friends, about the important things that nurses do, even if this means giving specific examples. In many cases, nurses literally keep patients alive and should not be modest in proclaiming this truth. It is also time for nurses to explain the nature of advanced education in nursing and to promulgate the results of nursing scholarship via all types of media on both local and national bases. A recent poll illustrated that the public wants professional nurses to care for them in hospitals ("Gallup finds," 1994). Let nursing give consumers the information they need to demand safe, professional nursing care. After all, "What cruel mistakes are sometimes made by benevolent men and women in matters of business about which they can do nothing and think they know a great deal" (Nightingale, 1860/1969, p. 134).

REFERENCES

American Nurses Association. (1993). *Position statement on registered nurse utilization of unlicensed assistive personnel.* Washington, DC: Author.

Barter, M., & Furmidge, M. L. (1994). Unlicensed assistive personnel: Issues relating to delegation and supervision. *Journal of Nursing Administration, 24*(4), 36–40.

Barter, M., McLaughlin, F., & Thomas, S. A. (1994). Use of unlicensed assistive personnel by hospitals. *Nursing Economics, 12*(2), 82–87.

Benner, P. (1984). *From novice to expert: Excellence and power in clinical nursing practice.* Menlo Park, CA: Addison-Wesley.

Donohue, M. P. (1985). *Nursing: The finest art.* St. Louis: C.V. Mosby.

Gallup finds most Americans opposed to RN staff cuts. (1994, August). *American Journal of Nursing,* p. 71.

Layoffs loom as Kaiser turns to 'multiskilled caregivers.' (1994, May). *American Journal of Nursing,* p. 77.

Manuel, P., & Alster, K. (1994). Unlicensed personnel: No cure for an ailing health care system. *Nursing and Health Care, 15*(1) 18–21.

Nightingale, F. (1969). *Notes on nursing: What it is, and what it is not.* New York: Dover Publications. (Original work published 1860)

Nutting, M. A., & Dock, L. L. (1907). *A history of nursing.* New York: G. P. Putnam's Sons.

Roberts, S. J. (1983). Oppressed group behavior: Implications for nursing. *Advances in Nursing Science, 5,* 21–30.

Schmieding, N. J. (1993). Nurse empowerment through context, structure, and process. *Journal of Professional Nursing, 9,* 239–245.

Striking at bargaining rights, court says RNs are supervisors. (1994, July). *American Journal of Nursing,* p. 67.

PART II

Interviews With Nursing Leaders

A

Elected and Appointed Public Officials

CHAPTER 12

Interview With Imogene King, RN, EdD, FAAN

Sandra B. Lewenson

Many nurses hold or have held public office and appointed policy positions; however, few people know this. The editor of this book, Harriet Feldman, and I began a search to uncover these nurses and "put a face"on each of them. In our book, *Nurses in the Political Arena: The Public Face of Nursing*, published by Springer Publishing, we identified and interviewed a number of these nurses and began to tell their stories. From our interviews we found that their nursing experience and expertise shaped their political ideas. Their backgrounds in nursing and interest in public service merged to create a synergy whereby they could become advocates for better health care in the legislative arena.

Learning who these nurses are was not an easy task. Lists kept by the American Nurses Association and the state nursing associations provided the bulk of the names; however, these records only revealed current office holders, so others were discovered by word of mouth. There is no central repository of this information, which means that the activities of politically-minded nurses are often not adequately reflected in nursing history.

While interviewing Imogene King for the Teachers College Centennial Celebration, I learned that this noted nursing theorist held public office in the 1970s. In 1975 she ran for and won the position of alderman for the small town where she lived outside of Chicago. In her brief tenure as an elected official, Dr. King dealt with

Note: Originally published in *Nursing Leadership Forum*, Vol. 4, No. 3, 2000. New York: Springer Publishing Company.

"dirty politics" during the campaign, brought several important issues to the table, and developed close ties with her constituents. During the interview, Dr. King provided a snapshot of her own educational background and the development of her interest in public service. She made it clear that it was extremely important for nurses to be politically active and she remains so today. She graciously agreed to a second interview where I posed the same questions used for *Nurses in the Political Arena: The Public Face of Nursing.* Although this interview highlights Dr. King's political story, the very background that shaped her theory development was what shaped her political goals and aspirations. The following are excerpts from the second interview with Dr. King.

Interviewer, Sandra B. Lewenson (SBL): Tell me about your background in nursing that led you to seek public office.

Imogene King (IK): It all started when World War II broke out in 1941. I was from a small town in Iowa and I had an uncle who was a surgeon and he said, because of the war, why didn't I think about going into nursing. I told him I never wanted to be a nurse. He convinced me that I should go to St. Louis into one of the two schools that he told me about. One had a 5-year program leading to a BS degree and the other, St. John's Hospital, led to a diploma. Five years seemed like a long time to me; it does to most people. So I chose the diploma school. I graduated in 1945, 1 month before the war was over.

Within a month I was back at a liberal arts college for girls. I was the nurse for the student boarders and was able to complete at least 36 to 38 hours of college work. It was a marvelous experience because it was still a boarding school and it was a finishing school for young ladies. We wore dinner dresses at night when we sat down for dinner, and we learned how to pour tea properly. I transferred to St. Louis University run by the Jesuits because the college did not award a professional degree. I was fortunate to be one of four women in the course. The Jesuits urged students to raise critical questions, and so it was a marvelous learning experience. In those days, the Jesuit universities required a minor in philosophy for a BS degree. You had to have a prerequisite course in logic before you could sign up for a philosophy course. Philosophy was my second area of interest and I've been into ethics ever since.

When I was at Teachers College, Columbia University in New York, I took one course in the history of baccalaureate education, so I was allowed into the Adelaide Nutting Special Collection. Another exciting experience I had while I was there, between 1959 and 1961, was meeting Isabel Stewart. Miss Stewart used to come for tea at least once a month, and she sat in the parlor. One day I was walking by, and I saw this lovely lady sitting there having a cup of tea, and I just walked in and she said: "Oh, good afternoon. I'm Isabel Stewart." I said, "I'm Imogene King, one of the students." I asked, "Would you mind if several of us come after you have your tea and just sit around and talk to you?" She said, "Not at all." So, I ran out and got three of my friends to join me in tea with Isabel Stewart. It was a wonderful experience.

SBL: How did your background in nursing influence some of the decisions you have made?

IK: When I finished the Bachelor of Science, one of the supervisors at the hospital school I was initially affiliated with asked me to come back and help her reorganize the nursing curriculum, which I did and then spent the next 10–12 years teaching in it and practicing at the hospital at the same time. This was in the days when teachers had to be able to practice before being allowed to teach. Now we have teachers who seem to be a little afraid to be in the clinical area. First, you are a teacher, then a practitioner. We believed you had to be a practitioner first, then a teacher. While I was there I went to Teachers College for a Master's degree and that's when I read about Mildred Montag's 5-year project in a community college program. I was fascinated with it because as a diploma grad during the war and because of the Cadet Nurse Corps, all of our didactic was given in 2 years, so that the cadets could go off some place else for practice in their senior year. I knew that you could do it in 2 years. A lot of people said we couldn't. I decided maybe I should get out of diploma education and get into the university system, and then I decided I couldn't do that without a doctoral degree. I don't know who gave me that idea. I thought I needed to go to New York and be taught by this wonderful woman. I applied and got accepted. I couldn't go the first year I was accepted because

I didn't have enough money saved. I went the second year and did really well the first semester, so I got one of the scholarships for the rest of it. But I finished in one calendar year and took one academic year for my doctorate. I told Dr. Montag that I had to go back and take care of my mother and that I needed to finish it in 2 years. She looked at me and said, "Try it!" She was a wonderful role model because she never coerced me in any way. In fact, once I walked past her office and she said, "Somebody told me you were going out to collect data. Do you think you should have a committee meeting first?" You talk about the right person for me. I wanted to move it and she didn't stop me. Then, I had a committee meeting and she facilitated that and put me on her calendar. Dr. Montag was wonderful.

SBL: When you ran for office, did you tell people about your nursing background?

IK: No, I didn't. This was in a suburban area of Chicago and I was teaching at Loyola University at the time and a lot of people in the community knew that I was teaching nursing students.

SBL: Tell me how you became involved in political life in the 1970s.

IK: I moved to Chicago to teach and I bought this condominium in suburban Chicago which was called Wood Dale, Illinois. This was a small community of 10,000 people, mostly from the middle to upper-middle class. I didn't know this when I bought the condo, but I was told that it was picketed while it was being built. Well, there were three pieces of property there and the real estate guy who owned it was going to build three condo buildings, but he died before they were finished. So the condo owners were in some kind of court case. They had already dug the foundation for a second building. The foundation was so deep that when the kids would come and ride their bikes down, the fire department had to come and get them out. I saw this one day when I was home and thought what a dangerous thing. So I said to the condominium board, "Does anyone want to go to City Hall with me? I think we need to talk to them about this." Nobody did and at that point,

I was made president of the condominium board. Nobody went with me, so I went by myself. I had never been to City Hall before and I went with my little speech. When it was time for citizens to speak, I said, "I live in this condominium and we have this deep hole dug out there and it is a real danger for the kids in the area. I wonder what I could do to get the City to fill the hole. I understand and see that you have this great building project and you have dump trucks picking up all this dirt and all you have to do is have them dump it in this hole." Simple solution. It wouldn't cost any money or anything. So the mayor looked at the city attorney sitting there and he said, "Why don't you go look to see if there is an ordinance that covers this." This didn't make sense to me. I waited and after a half-hour this attorney came back and the mayor asked, "What did you find?" The only thing he could find was a noise ordinance. My mouth opened and I said, "That doesn't fit this situation."

The mayor thanked me for coming. I went home, but before I did I looked in at that City Council and they were all men sitting there. I wasn't impressed by the meeting and the kinds of issues they were discussing. Then I went out and dug out some information about the community. They had two problems. The first was that they were in debt and couldn't get a credit rating; and the second was that they had problems with their police force.

I was driving to work about a week later and I stopped at this light and the mayor's car was next to me. So I rolled down my window and said, "Mr. Mayor, how are you? I'm waiting to hear from you. By the way, how do you get on the city committee? I think since I heard about the financial problem, I would like to be on your Finance Committee." The mayor told me to call his daughter. I called and she said that her father thought that I ought to run for office. "Well," I said "I really want to be on the Finance Committee because I think I can help you get out of debt." She said we would talk with him again. She called me later to tell me that she had my ward all figured out. She invited me to meet her and told me that I should run for alderman. I went to our vice president at the university and I asked if it was appropriate for me to run. Could I do something like this? The vice president said, "Oh, do it." It was 1975 and I ran for office. I was the first woman to run in that community.

SBL: Tell me about the campaign, I understand that you had to overcome some "dirty" politics.

IK: The Sunday before the Tuesday election, a "dirty" White Paper went out about me. Two of the guys who sat on that Council did not like me, obviously, and so they had put out this information. It was interesting that I was only a fairly new home owner in that community. People called me to react to this. These men had a reputation for nasty politics and for running people out of town. People in my ward got together and wrote up a document after they had asked me some questions about these nasty comments. They had the Boy Scouts pass this response around to my ward the night before the election. This was really an interesting political experience for me. I got elected with an overwhelming majority of votes.

The most interesting thing was that the polling place was right next door to our condo, so I went to vote early that morning and here were the two aldermen from each area. The alderman that I would work with if I got elected was standing there. The first thing he said was he didn't have a thing to do with that White Paper. I said, "Who are you?" He gave me his name and I said, "Well, I don't know you so why would you know about the White Paper." So, I figured he was part of it. At the first two meetings, he had two women in the audience who said, "We don't know where our alderman is because we call her and she's never at home." I said, "I'm sorry, but I do work." The next week that we had a meeting, the same two women came saying the same thing. In the meantime, I checked them out and they weren't even in my ward. So I said, "I'm sorry ladies, but I think you're calling the wrong alderman because I understand that from where you live, you are not in my ward. So there wouldn't be much I could do to help you unless it's a city-wide problem." Well, you know, they walked right out, embarrassed. Of course, I'm sitting next to the alderman, and I said, "Tony, you don't know me very well, but you pull a dirty trick like this one more time, and you're going to go out the back door. I'm here as an honest citizen and I'm just going to try to help this city . . . we need to work together." Well, from then on, it was a little easier until one night he came and he was bit befuddled, and I looked at him and said, "What's the matter?" He told me his father was very ill in the hospital. Well, my nursing experience came out and I said, "Tell me about it, and maybe I can explain some things to you." So, we had this nice conversation and he said, "I can't thank you enough, you really filled me in." I said, "That's why I'm here."

Six months after my election as alderman, I was appointed to Chairman of the Finance Committee. Did I have fun! I got the bond passed, passed the utility tax, and spread the word to the whole community. Here again the Boy Scouts carried our messages to everybody in the community. So we got out of debt in a year and a half. Of course, the people came when they found out that we passed the utility tax. It didn't cost any homeowner more than $3 for the year, the way we figured it. But it was just wonderful. Then I got to the police department, because one of our young policeman had a coronary. So I went to the chief and said, "We're going to get a health plan started here. . . . We're going to exercise and do the things that prevent this from happening." They finally decided that a nurse was a smart decision-maker who could solve problems.

SBL: What were some of the other issues you brought to the Council?

IK: I went to work on the building code because it had been amended so much that you couldn't read it. Only one guy, one of the staff, could make sense out of it and he had a conflict. Anyway, I said, let's set up a Citizen's Committee. So I set it up just before I left office and the building code was changed to be a performance code that was absolutely beautiful. Those are the little things I did.

SBL: The people saw you differently because you were a nurse?

IK: I don't think so, but you know what was interesting? When I came to my first meeting, the sign in front of me read Miss Imogene King. There was an alderman who was a dentist and his sign identified him as "doctor." So I went to the City Clerk and explained if the dentist was referred to as doctor, then I wanted a new sign made for the next meeting that included the title doctor. I got a new sign at the next meeting. I think we have to demand the respect that we deserve. I always do that. First you have to respect me as a person, then you respect me as a nurse.

SBL: What impact have you had on the political process and some of the outcomes?

IK: We had a new performance building code. We were out of debt and we built a contingency fund so the city could do some nice things for the city. The personnel policies were corrected so that the head honcho of the department made a little more money than the next highest paid person. I go to the grocery store and the women who would see me would walk up to me and say, "You ought to run for senator, because the present senator doesn't like women." If I had been a little younger and the snow in Chicago not so unpleasant, I think I would have stayed and probably ran.

SBL: What made you leave Chicago and your political base?

IK: There were so many snows in Chicago that year and I was 57 years old and I thought, I don't need this. I need to go to Florida and work in the health care system. I can learn the system and then retire there, because I knew I wanted to retire in Florida to play golf. And that's what I did. But I wanted to work in the system before I settled here; and I'm glad I did, because I got to know the medical system and the health care system.

SBL: Have you stayed active in politics since your experience as alderman?

IK: I've always been active. I believe that if the Congress and Senate don't hear from us, then we don't have a leg to stand on in terms of anything that goes on in society and in terms of our laws. I always called and made an appointment and introduced myself whenever I moved to a new area. I'll tell you about my experience in Florida. When I moved to St. Petersburg I got a new legislator, so I called his office and said I would like to make an appointment. I use "Doctor" when I'm doing this. Since I just moved to the area and he was my legislator, I would really like to talk to him. I was being put off, of course. I know they protect these people. I told them a little about what I was doing and in a few minutes was asked what day I would like to meet him. I made an appointment and while sitting in his office, I noticed all these plaques in the other office and learned he was a practicing chiropractor. That gave me some information about him, so when I met him I told him I was a nurse and that I had warm feelings toward chiropractors because I had worked with one earlier in my career. I offered my help if he needed information about nursing and told him and that I wanted to be his resource person. He said, "That's wonderful, I never had anybody do that before."

During this last legislative session, I called him before the session began to give him some feedback on three health-related bills. I had found out that he was Chairman of the Health Committee. I left a message with his secretary that I wanted him to vote "yes" and could he call me if he needed more information. On his way to Tallahassee on Saturday morning, I got a call from him. I thought, isn't that kind of neat! That's the kind of relationship we should be building. They respect you, and if you say you're going to give them information, you do.

SBL: What have you learned in your many years of being politically active?

IK: When I was in Washington I learned that the Administrative Assistant, at least in Congress, is the key person you want to get to, because you can't always talk to the elected officials. They are too busy, but the administrative assistant knows all of the constituents and that's how you get through. I believe that politics is power. Power is the energy that helps us achieve those goals and the politicians have power. I never send a nasty note or letter or make a nasty phone call. Everything I do with the politicians is in a normal tone of voice and a positive statement about something. Or I ask them to please look at this and I hope they won't vote for it, because these are the consequences if they do. I always give some rationale for why I'm calling. The minute you're nasty, you are considered a crank, and they really don't hear you after that; and that's just human nature.

SBL: How did you develop some of your political skills?

IK: None of my skills, except my nursing skills, has been quite purposeful. Probably my skills stem from my undergraduate work at St. Louis when we had to, in philosophy, raise our voices about an issue; we had to give a rationale, and that's tough stuff when you are defending a philosophical position against philosophers. The whole idea of critical thinking and logical reasoning was part of that educational process, but you had to defend your position. That's a skill that a lot of people I think don't ever learn. My diploma school made me an excellent nurse, no doubt about it. There too, I think, we were taught to think through things. When we left that school, we were highly skilled in every skill that a nurse needed to have, including the thinking skills.

SBL: How did you think you interfaced with the public when you held office?

IK: It was fun. It was a small community and I met people in the grocery store. We chatted and if they had a complaint, I would take it to the Council. In fact, those women said that they would elect me to anything I wanted to run for or I went around for. So, indirectly or directly I was getting kudos from the people in the community.

SBL: What advice would you give someone now in terms of running for office, or holding an appointed position?

IK: When I did this I was very naive. I would suggest that the person first get together with people who had run committees and campaigns and find out what it is, get down to the grass roots and find out what a campaign is really all about. Then decide why you want to run for office, what you want to bring to it, what you want to do, what kind of decisions should be made that are not being made, because you give an awful lot of your time and energy if you are really committed. That's what I would do—learn how a campaign is run. I'd get information, then I make the decision if I want to do it, and then I would set up a committee.

Dr. King ran for and held public office at a time when few women had the opportunity to do so. It was during the politically turbulent 1970s when the women's movement encouraged women to enter careers typically dominated by men, like medicine, and abandon more traditional careers for women, like nursing. Well-educated and working in the academic arena, Dr. King questioned a potential health hazard in her community and challenged the political status quo. She found support from many in her community but also had to deal with what she called "dirty politics." People questioned her role as a working woman and attempted to discredit her.

Dr. King met the challenges while in office and was able to make significant changes in her community. During the interview she noted several times that if she had been younger, she might have run for senator. Dr. King continues to be engaged in politics and has recently been reelected to serve on the Board of the Florida Nurses Association. She envisions a task force that would look at the health care system in the state of Florida and hopes to garner support from the Florida Nurses Association and the Governor. Like the many other nurses we interviewed for *Nurses in the Political Arena: The Public Face of Nursing*, Dr. King recognizes the link between politics and health care and has been a strong advocate for and a model of political involvement for nurses. Though widely acclaimed for her work in theory development, Dr. King's work in politics equally serves the advancement of nursing.

CHAPTER 13

Interview With Diane O. McGivern, RN, PhD, FAAN

Barbara Stevens Barnum

> *Interviewer, Barbara Stevens Barnum (BB):* We are very fortunate in New York State to have a major nurse leader serving in a highly important and visible political position on the Board of Regents. Diane, would you give our readers your professional background before we get into your role on the Board?
>
> Diane O. McGivern (DM): I'm Head of the Division of Nursing at New York University (NYU) here in New York City. The Division was established in 1929 as part of the School of Education and we have three levels of instruction in the Nursing Division: baccalaureate, master's, and doctoral. We have 33 full-time nursing faculty and approximately 120 part-time faculty, and we serve about 1,000 students. We're very much a part of the mission of NYU, which is a private university in the public service, so we're very involved with community-based practice and meeting the needs of the urban underserved population.

> *BB:* Not all states have a body equivalent to our Board of Regents. Would you describe the Board's function for our readers?
>
> DM: The Board of Regents is a policy-making body that oversees the Department of Education in New York State. It was

Note: Originally published in *Nursing Leadership Forum,* Vol. 3, No. 4, 1998. New York: Springer Publishing Company.

established after the revolutionary war in order to begin to rebuild higher education in the state. At that time, higher education resided in one institution, Kings College, which is now Columbia University. The legislative mandate for the Board of Regents grew over the years, adding considerably to the scope of its responsibility. Although it started over-seeing higher education, the mandate quickly encompassed elementary and secondary education as well. Today, the scope of responsibility includes all of education from birth through university, including life-long learning. The licensed profes-sions, of which there are now 38 in New York, were included as were various cultural institutions which include museums, libraries, and historical societies. The mandate also includes services to individuals with disabilities, all together, a very broad sweep of responsibilities. I believe New York State is the only state where that scope of responsibility exists within one policy-making body. The advantage is that the connect-edness between all of these areas becomes part of the broad panorama. Connections can be made and the resources of one area can be used by another.

It's also different in another respect: the Governor has no direct appointing responsibility for the State Education Department. The Board of Regents was in fact created for just that reason, as a buffer against the political pressures that affect public education. The members of the Board of Regents are elected by the combined legislature. In turn, the Board of Regents recruits and appoints the Commissioner of Education. Therefore this Commissioner is the only one in New York State who is not appointed by the Governor, although the Commissioner and Board of Regents work col-laboratively with the Governor.

BB: You say that the Board of Regents is not accountable to the Governor. Do you see that as good or not so good?

DM: This Governor has called for the dissolution of the Board of Regents in the past, but he's somewhat muted about that now. He has adopted much of our educational agenda in the last 2 years as his own. It means that the new Commissioner and our Chancellor have been very aggressive in pursuing better relationships with the Governor. There are also a num-

ber of other considerations. New York City is very different
from Upstate New York. It is almost a different region in terms
of legislative thinking and in terms of which issues are hot.
Not that the issues are different, but the sheer density of them
in the city makes it seem like a different scenario downstate.

Education is also heavily politicized for other reasons.
Everyone in the state has a stake in it, not only because they
have children or grandchildren. The economy of the state
depends on well educated people. Everyone pays taxes, and
there's a close relationship in everyone's mind between their
tax burden and the education system. I'm not sure people
understand what the demands are in public education.
Because public education is fairly insulated—in the sense that
the general public doesn't walk into a school—the public's
personal memories of going to school color what they think
is operating. For example, people are very surprised to find
that practically no school has its own school nurse, that children are not making trips to the dentist, or that many children don't have access to school trips because of the
bureaucratic morass of dealing with bus schedules. They would
be surprised to see that the interiors of many buildings pose
real health hazards. There are buildings where there has been
water damage resulting in environmental hazards. People are
simply not aware, yet they feel empowered to speak about
education.

Public higher education is another issue. It's politicized in
the sense that we have a large city education system and a
large state education system, each with their own agendas.
The strong private sector also has its agenda. Each has a set
of supporters as well. Clearly, it is challenging to be dealing
with these diverse populations.

BB: Do the schools see the Board of Regents as interfering or
as their advocate?

DM: Teachers and administrators on the building level have
their own perspectives. One of the things the Board has tried
to do is to become more visible to the educators and people
in the community. Some people think of us as the state, a distant generator of policies, not necessarily helpful. Others are
very engaged in the Board of Regents' work. There are hun-

dreds and thousands of teachers, superintendents, principals, and college presidents involved in various advisory groups—policy recommending groups. There's a broad range. There's a real effort on the part of the Board to understand what people are thinking. We want to know, what is the experience in the field as a result of the policy the Regents' make? A lot of discussion takes place with the community and individuals. We want to see what policies are working, what issues need to be addressed. No matter who you are (teacher, principal, superintendent), you are somewhat reserved about talking about all the things you are dealing with when someone in a policy making role drops in on you. It's very heartening to go to the schools and see effective learning taking place.

One of the things I've tried to talk about when I talk to other nurses is the need to be more engaged in the mission of education. Ultimately, that is self-serving, particularly for those of us in nursing. We want to see our profession recruit well-educated, well-prepared individuals. We will not be able to recruit the population we need if we do not understand and attend to the quality of elementary and secondary education. I visit schools where there is no science program because there's no water. We know the students aren't prepared to think about careers related to science technology. They can't possibly be prepared for nursing careers. So we have a vested interest in being advocates for education improvement. We also have a vested interest in health services for children. Specialty nursing groups such as school nurses and nurse practitioners demonstrate that, but it really should be a broader based commitment.

BB: How did you decide to put yourself forward as a candidate for the Board?

DM: In 1987–88, there was a great deal of publicity about the Board of Regents in our local paper because our representative from Staten Island, the 2nd district, had decided not to run. I read the information and thought, *Well that's something I have had experience with, especially higher education, accreditation, and professional practice.* In a tremendous burst of naivety, I thought, *That looks interesting, I think I'll look into it.* A neighbor who was a member of the assembly was very interested in nominating me. The seat for the 2nd judicial district had, interestingly enough, been held by a physician, and so, for at least as long as my predecessors held the position, it became known as the physician's seat. That label was strange because it's a lay board, with no designation of any seat. But the physician's seat had become a tradition.

I completed the interviews. The selection process is a whole series of interviews and public forums in which people are questioned by members of the Education Committees and others on various topics. I went back and forth to Albany for interviews numerous times: it was reasonably stressful. They were still looking for a physician, and every physician I knew was brought up to Albany. Ultimately, a cardiothoracic surgeon was selected, but he had not been in good health and was only able to serve 3 years of his term. When the position became vacant again, my husband said, "Would you want to try that again?" I said, "I don't think I want to go through that again." But another member of the assembly called and asked if I were willing to be a candidate. Fortunately, the 3-year interim was brief enough that they remembered my previous interviews. The issues had changed somewhat but not completely. In the initial interviews the hot issues had been: the AIDS curriculum, condom distribution, and the multicultural curriculum and what that meant. The briefer, second set of interviews went well and ultimately I was elected. That was in March 1991.

BB: What functions did you perform on the Board?

DM: When I started on the Board, I was appointed to the Professional Practice Committee, the Elementary and Secondary Education Committee, and the Committee on Services to Individuals With Disability. I was reelected to a second term on my own, and then in 1998, I was elected Vice Chancellor of the Board.

I've spent a lot of time working on special education in New York City, about which a great deal had been written and about which a great deal needs to be done. Most recently, I've cochaired the Committee on the Task Force on Teaching, which produced a set of recommendations and reports that was voted on by the Board. This work had to do with teacher preparation and certification around the state. That was important for several reasons. First, we spent the last 8 or 9 years looking at improving standards for elementary and secondary education. Clearly, not only were higher content standards needed, but also more rigorous testing standards and more rigorous graduation requirements, including passing Regents' examinations to get a high school diploma. The other side of that equation, of course, is that, if you have higher standards for children, you have to have teachers who are equipped to teach to those standards.

We spent an inordinate amount of time looking at this topic. In the 2 years it took us to look at what was actually going on, several things became very clear. One was the disparity in performance among children across the state as well as the discrepancy among teachers. Another discovery was the wide range of quality and resources in teacher preparation programs. There are about 120 programs of teacher education in the state, and one of the significant findings was that in about one fourth to one third of all teacher programs, only 30% of their graduates were able to pass one or more of the certification examinations. Of particular concern in New York City was the fact that youngsters in the public schools take as teaching role models the teachers they have. They themselves then enter teacher preparation programs which are not of the highest expectations. They then cycle back into the city public school system, creating an unfortunate cycle of modest performance expectations. Several of the recommendations included that teacher preparation programs be accredited, and in teacher preparation programs, 80% of the graduates must pass the state examination or they will be subject to deregistration. We also, on the other side, needed to look at providing incentives for people to choose teaching as a career in addition to urging colleges and universities to improve their programs and to create more innovative programs.

Before our recommendations there were no professional development requirements for currently practicing teachers. There is now a requirement of 175 hours in a 5-year period and a number of other recommendations that affect systems and will assure competency.

BB: How does your service on the Board connect to nursing?

DM: People are pleased that there is a nurse on the Board of Regents after 215 years of its existence, and I am pleased to be known as a nurse on the Board. Simply by being in the place, you raise people's consciousness. Very often when people give examples about the professions or educational preparation, they'll include nursing in their examples because they are looking right at me. It reminds them that nursing is very much connected with what the Board does.

I find a great deal of similarity between elementary and secondary education and nursing education, for obvious reasons. I think health defined in the broadest possible way includes things like becoming a competent learner. Certainly in public policy, health is defined broadly to include education, housing, and adequate nutrition. Nursing has that same perspective on health. Many of the issues pertinent to elementary, secondary, and higher education have to do with the integration of services that allow people to take advantage of education. Most of us are quite familiar with the need for children to be healthy in order to be ready to learn. We're concerned about access to primary care, to school-based health services; we're aware of the severe deficit of mental health services for children, particularly in underserved areas. Those are issues that have always been the domain of nursing. We are very aware that new populations coming to New York State have not always had any exposure to organized state services. Children come here never having had health services, frequently living in marginal housing. All of those factors create real deficits. The issues are quite central to nursing.

BB: Has your experience with nursing's accreditation processes and state evaluations helped you?

DM: Very much so. So much of what we do in nursing is very far ahead of what other professions are currently practicing. Let me give you just a few examples. The accreditation of our programs, whether the criteria are sufficiently rigorous or not, whether they are focused on outcomes or not, is far and away superior to what we see in other professional disciplines. The expectations about practice, the integration of our code of ethics in practice, our understanding of the place of client, are all so established in our minds that we don't recognize that we are in a different place from other professions. In looking at teacher preparation and their professional practice, I was surprised to find that accreditation was not an expectation, that peer review and evaluation were not as deeply imbedded in professional practice of teaching as they are for nursing. We take for granted our analytic approach to things, our "can do" attitude, and our ability to take action. When we step outside of the nursing profession and get involved in some of the other professions, we are surprised to find things quite different.

BB: Are there any times when you think that your influence has been of special importance on issues acted on by the Board?

DM: Every Board member feels that he or she has a significant influence on the content and course of the discussion. The Board of Regents, by virtue of having 16 members, each with particular expertise, can make better policy than any one individual. Each Board member also has a particular area of interest, so one is assigned to relevant work. I have been fortunate enough to be assigned to the professional practice arena where we have looked at problems like the environmental impact on practice, certain disciplinary problems, and the effects of corporatization on practice.

Some of the other disciplines also work in an environment that has changed radically in the past few years, for example, pharmacy practice or accounting. There are many things to consider concerning the corporatization of practice, whether you are considering a whole range of disciplinary cases or just one. Several years ago, for example, we looked at environmental factors and medication errors. The results of that survey showed that nurses made more errors when they were working in institutions where overtime was required, when they felt coerced into working more than one shift, or where there was very little supervision and very little orientation. These results were not surprising; you could easily demonstrate a pattern of poor institutional practices. Understanding the environment in which these people were practicing was something I brought to the Board.

BB: How long does one serve as a Regent?

DM: When the Board was created, people were appointed for lifetime. Since then, the length of the appointment has been continuously reduced. Currently the appointment is 5 years. When I started, it was 7. It's always interesting, for good reasons and bad, when the legislature gets upset about education in the state, and then decreases the term of the Board members. But 5 years is probably a reasonable term. The other thing that has changed is that people tended to be reelected in the past. Some would be on the Board for 15 to 25 years. That has changed rather dramatically because the legislators demand that the Board be more active. There has been quite a turnover in Board membership. The new Chancellor, Carl Hayden, has created also a high level of expectation for being proactive. In my case, I completed 4 years of the surgeon's term and was reelected. My reelected term will end in the year 2000.

BB: Will you run again?

DM: It's hard to tell. Serving on the Board is equivalent to another full-time job. We meet 11 times a year, once a month for 2 1/2 days. All of the other Board obligations can sometimes add 2 other days a week. That's a fairly significant responsibility. Added to that, there are some members who spend even more time in Board activities. Some people assume that this is a paid position and are disappointed to find it is not. But it is certainly interesting; you learn as much as you give to Board discussions. That's terrific. Whether to run again is not something I want to make a decision about right now. So much changes from year to year, and I think shorter terms are better in the long run for the Board.

BB: Do you anticipate taking any other public arena jobs?

DM: I think you always find a reason to participate in the public arena without actually planning for it. Years ago, when I was a Robert Wood Johnson Health Policy Fellow, there were expectations about how you would use that expertise. Some people did in ways that were clearly connected. I think that my tenure on the Board of Regents draws on that year spent in Washington. What I learned there was very new for me. So it all comes together. Certainly, my position at New York University is also very exciting. There are a lot of opportunities here, and it's a matter of having the time and energy to pursue them.

BB: We've talked about what your appointment has done for nursing and the public, but what has it done for you personally?

DM: It's very enriching to have an opportunity to learn in great detail issues and circumstances that you would never have been exposed to otherwise. I know a great deal about a lot of educational issues and about the people who are advocating for issues, people whom I would never have met in other forums. Throughout the city there are strong grass root advocacy groups, people who are trying to improve education, largely prompted by their own children's entry into the system. And they're dealing at the school level, especially women who are educating themselves about public education and advocating for education against tremendous counter pressures not to get involved in what some school schools officials feel is their turf.

And, of course, you meet wonderful people who are professionals in the system. You see the issues they have to deal with—a significant set of issues, particularly in the urban setting, but in the rural settings as well. One gets a wonderful panorama of the whole issue of the school environment and the environment immediately surrounding the schools, the bureaucratic structure that makes it difficult for some of the leadership, and the whole range of social issues that impact on the children that it is serving.

One learns the difficulty of teaching without appropriate services. Teachers often are not only responsible for teaching, but also for managing some issues that are outside their professional preparation. Those are tremendously important things to address. It's exciting to meet people who are successfully counteracting all of that, people who are in various policy or advocacy organizations, who are extraordinarily well versed in some of the issues like the legal aspects of the special education system. Some people have spent their lives advocating for these rights. Having the opportunity to meet and learn from these people is one of the greatest benefits of being a Board member.

BB: It sounds like a challenging and rewarding role. The nursing profession has clearly benefited by your representation on this prestigious policy-making body.

B

Caregivers

CHAPTER 14

Interview With Eugene Sawicki, RN, EdD, MDiv, JCL: When the Nurse Is a Priest

Barbara Stevens Barnum

Dr. Sawicki was interviewed by Barbara Stevens Barnum at Our Lady of Vilnius Lithuanian Catholic Church in lower Manhattan, where he serves as priest and administrator.

> *Interviewer, Barbara Stevens Barnum (BB):* Dr. Sawicki, you have the unique distinction of being both a doctorally prepared nurse and a priest. I know that you completed your EdD in nursing before becoming a priest, but which of these two careers came first in your interest?
>
> Eugene Sawicki (ES): My first interest was to be a priest; I always wanted to be a priest, but I never saw it as "either-or." I remember saying to myself as a youth, "Why can't I be priestly and practice another profession at the same time?" I wanted to combine both. To be priestly is to practice a vocation, to be a protector and a preserver. To be an encourager, nurse, and healer is also to do something of the priestly work.
>
> *BB:* You wanted to combine working and the priesthood?
>
> ES: The ideal was of a worker priest, that is, a priest with a special mission, a priest who has a dual career. The priesthood for me is primary, but the exercise of it is not limited to the

---

Note: Originally published in *Nursing Leadership Forum*, Vol. 1, No. 3, 1995. New York: Springer Publishing Company.

traditional role, and it can be exercised in a nontraditional setting. Paul was a tent maker. To be a nurse is not antithetical to the priesthood. Among the working people, among the sick, the nurses and the caretakers are the visible presence of God. The mystery we call God should be at the workplace as well as in the church on the weekend. We should be encouraged to be aware of the mystery in which we live at all times, not only during the formally religious time once week.

BB: You were a nurse before you were a priest. When you first became a priest, was there any role confusion or adjustment? Was it difficult to switch from one identity to the other?

ES: Before I was a priest, I was a nurse, but I considered the nurse role that of healer, very much akin to the priesthood— for me at least. For instance, I would bless the medicine before I gave it. Nobody would see it, but it's a way of potentiating the medicine. Or I would bless the patients when I would pray for them or over them. That was as a nurse.

Now that I'm a priest, I can do it overtly. There can be a spiritual interchange between them and me. I can anoint them with holy oils, pray over them, bring them the Eucharist, and do the things that the priest does as well as doing the nursing part. Of course, there's a certain practical conflict, and you can't always do two things at once. Sometimes you can: When you're taking care of a patient, you can also be praying over him and asking God to help the healing process. As a Catholic priest, I believe the dimension of mystery is accentuated for me. When people know I'm both a priest and a nurse, it breaks down their ordinary categories and stretches their minds.

BB: Have you done active nursing since becoming a priest?

ES: Yes, when I go to visit the patients, the flock, the old people, when I bring holy communion to them, I have an awareness of their physical and psychological needs as well as the theological ones. I go to heal the whole person. The theological is one aspect of the person. As a priest, I go in there to anoint them, bless them, perhaps to bring holy communion to their homes. Yet I automatically do a nursing assessment. In that sense I do nursing even though I don't get paid for it. I don't do formal nursing, but I do nursing continually because our education and instinct is to be thinking, assessing, and paying attention to the patient. What do they need? What will help them? Nor is a true nurse limited to the physical.

BB: So your nursing background comes into play instinctively?

ES: Not just instinctively but through learning, through education.

BB: Do people hold different expectations of you when they know you are also a nurse? Does it affect the way people relate to you?

ES: It does in many cases. When you talk to patients only as a priest, they never talk about anything physical. They figure you wouldn't understand. When they find out I'm a nurse, they open up: "This hurts, that hurts. Why is this happening?" I'm able to do more; my role is expanded. I don't see why roles can't be expanded for other priests as well. Of course, you can reverse this perspective and ask why the spiritual dimension of nursing can't be extended. I think that is changing, however, and it is generally expanding.

BB: You see a spiritual element being added to nursing?

ES: The whole universe is drifting from the material to the spiritual, from the physical to the energetic, from the practical to the psychic, from matter to energy. So it is not surprising that there is a renewed spiritual interest. Naturally, this trend would show itself in nursing, which is always attuned to the person and groups of people. If I am with old people, for example, teaching them health care, I don't limit myself to clinical aspects like, "What do you do with your colostomy?" I become aware, for example, of their need to pray, their need to be aware of the mysterious presence of God. I help them confront their dying, their immortality, and their need to make sense of where they are now. The spiritual dimension is not to be eschewed in the interest of being clinical.

BB: There certainly is more in the literature on spiritual aspects of nursing recently. What ought to be taught to a nurse in relation to spirituality?

ES: As long as nurses are going to care for a whole person, they have to pay attention to the theological needs of the person, whether the person is young or old. The way people look at spirituality, at the life of man with God, is going to vary. The young person isn't aware of the mystery of God the way an old person is. The child is not aware of God like a middle-aged person is. If the nurse is going to approach patients on the entire age spectrum, he must be aware of each person's theological dimension. People should learn the theological dimension at their mothers' knees. They should be taught to pray. Why are they here? Where are they going? These questions are important. Colleges of nursing should prepare persons for these ideas. They must if the nurse is to take care of the whole person. How can you treat one leg and not the other? One aspect of the personality and not the other?

There is a movement toward the spiritual and the psychic worldwide at many levels. It certainly is reflected in the schools of nursing where people are being encouraged to consider what it means to be human. What is the mystery of the universe? Does it affect us?

This should be apart of the course work. A truly intellectual approach should consider the spiritual. Others say it's irrelevant, that church and state should be separate, and spirituality has nothing to do with the real world. It's theoretical and abstract, they say; we must concentrate on the concrete; don't bother us with the religious stuff. Well, their position is unexamined; their presuppositions underdeveloped.

BB: We've talked about how you've combined being a priest and a nurse. Outside of those practicalities, has the fact that you're a nurse made you a better priest?

ES: Has nursing helped me be a better priest? Of course it has, by making me attentive to the practical in living. It's easy for the theoretician or the philosopher to lose touch. Einstein said that every scientist should be a shoemaker. I don't see why every priest can't be something else—a full-time priest but at the same time having a concentration in another field as well.

BB: Have you ever had an occasion when the two careers have come into conflict?

ES: No. I can imagine cases where it could happen, but I haven't had one. Obviously, there are issues where treatments conflict with religious beliefs. These have been discussed traditionally in nursing programs; abortion and euthanasia come to mind. But the more common problems may be more subtle. I can imagine a conflict might come up for a nurse administrator where the people are viewed as secondary to goals of the organization. In that situation, the priestly part of me would say, "Wait a minute. The Catholic tradition says that people are not here to be pawns. We're not here to help other people make money and to suffer inconveniences to increase somebody else's profit margin." Such a situation might come up in nursing administration.

BB: I hope you continue to be fortunate in not having such conflicts. Do some people come to you with different kinds of problems because of your being both priest and nurse?

ES: Many people don't know I'm both. When I'm acting as a nurse, I don't go out of my way to inform them. If there's a reason to tell them I'm a priest, I tell them. Otherwise I don't. And when I'm being a priest, I don't ordinarily talk about myself. I'll tell them I'm a nurse only if it comes up somehow. Only rarely will I say, "Look, I'm a doctorally prepared nurse."

Sometimes it surprises people who know me only in one context or the other. This occurred once when I was teaching emergency procedures for student teachers, therapeutic recreation counselors, and special education teachers at Mercy College to prepare them to handle unusual situations. Because I was in the nursing role, I wore civilian clothes to teach. After the course was over, at the last class, I came in wearing my Roman collar. The students were shocked. "We would never have said the things we did if we thought you were a priest," they said. I was surprised to hear that, surprised to hear that they'd be reluctant to speak.

BB: Do you ever think about enhancing your nursing practice skills?

ES: Sure. When my situation changes, I may have to concentrate on one clinical area, but I hope not to be limited to one area. Like any nurse, I need constant updating. I need supervision; I need to be with people who can teach me.

BB: It sounds like you don't ever intend to say you "used to be a nurse."

ES: Never. Once a nurse, always a nurse; it's a mark that appears on the soul. I know that some feel they're no longer nurses because they're not in formal paid practice, but any woman who is a nurse and raises a family will tell you that she takes care of the whole neighborhood as well. I use my nursing all the time. Nursing and the priesthood share many things. They both call for healing at the seven different levels of personhood. You are constantly calling upon what you know: assessing, intervening, and calling on all your resources.

BB: Seven different levels? Is that a construct from religion or nursing? What do you mean by those levels?

ES: Seeing the personality as having seven dimensions is reflected in various philosophical systems, in Thomistic-Aristotelian philosophy, for example, where things are highly schematized. It is a theological approach in many different traditions.

The seven levels include the theological, the philosophical, the psychological, the sociological, the economic, the aesthetic, and the physical. In the theological dimension, we think about God and where we're going. The philosophical dimension asks the questions of existence. What does it mean to be alive? Do we have immortality? What's going on around me, within me, outside me? How do I know that I can know—epistemology—philosophical aspects. The psychological dimension looks at people as individuals. How does the person grow and develop? What component of his being is nature, what is nurture? What can be done to promote psychological health? The sociological dimension looks at man as part of the group. Is the group more important than the individual? Does the group have an identity? Is it homogenous? How do I relate to family and friends?

The economic dimension is practical: Do I sell my soul in my effort to make money? Is it the primary goal? Is my remuneration sufficient for my happiness? The aesthetic dimension asks, what is beauty? Is it important to have beauty around me? Is there beauty in people? In objects? In nature? Is it important to me? Am I conscious of beauty? The aesthetic dimension can be enhanced by our education. We're attracted to beauty. We need loveliness, balance, and symmetry.

For me, the physical dimension comes from nursing. In nursing you learn the intricacy of body, the complexity of the organism, the physical level of being. What am I? Am I more than the sum of my parts? What are my parts? What does it mean to be human? What is the endocrine influence on my behavior? The physical is an essential part of the theological. Each part is an essential part of the other. You can't look at any aspect in isolation. They must be integrated.

BB: It sounds like a concept that would work for nursing as well as theology.

ES: As a matter of fact, when I was nursing at Bellevue, they taught this. I just use it as a way to lend order to the inquiring mind, whether a priest, a student nurse, or an administrator. It's a paradigm that lends order so that you can deal with the mystery of personhood. You must have order first before you can deal with apparent disorder and mystery. But positive confusion is good: Out of confusion comes a higher level of orderliness. It is like that with mystery. Mystery is not a case of ignorance; it's knowing so much you see how much you don't know. Mystery is built on knowledge, and human beings are mysterious.

Nursing is mysterious. How do we heal in spite of ourselves? What does it mean when a patient gets much better? Is it because you prayed over him? Or is your caring for him a form of prayer—the transmission of love energy? I believe it is the transmission of very high frequency electromagnetic waves that brings about a realignment in the other person's wave—a phenomenon which we call healing because we can see its measurable effect.

So much of healing, living, and nursing is mysterious. Certainly being a priest is mysterious. Of any type of healing, we can ask: Do we do it? Does God do it? Is it natural to us? These things give us a sense of awe and respect for our patients, for our teachers, and for each other. We should marvel at the people around us. For the nurse, the patient is the special focus.

BB: Dr. Sawicki, you certainly have blended these two careers in such a consistent pattern that they seem natural together. Yet, in truth, the combination is quite extraordinary. I certainly don't know any other nurses who are priests.

ES: I've heard of a couple of priests with RNs in the United States. There's a brother with a doctorate in nursing, but no other priests to my knowledge. The other priests who are nurses aren't doctorally prepared.

BB: Do any extra duties fall your way because you're a doctorally prepared nurse?

ES: That's why I ended up representing the Archdiocese of New York at the United Nations for the International Catholic Nurses, a nongovernmental organization (NGO) of the United Nations. These groups do most of the nondiplomatic work of the UN, the actual day-by-day healing, reconstructing, revivifying of countries and people. There are many such groups, for example, the Peace Adjusters Group, the International Catholic Nurses Group, Pax Christi, and Caritas International. Every 4 years the UN International Catholic Nurses and Medical Workers hold a worldwide conference. This group is a Vatican organization as well.

In 1990, New York was chosen as the site for the congress. Since one of the topics chosen was "Ethics and Decision-Making," the Vatican and Archdiocese of New York requested that the speaker be a priest. The nurses, on the other hand, wanted to hear from a nurse, and all desired the speaker to be doctorally prepared. Father-Doctor-Nurse Sawicki fell into that slot, so I delivered the address.

BB: Thank you so much, Dr. Sawicki. I think your answers will give our readers much to reflect on.

In addition to his degrees in nursing, Dr. Sawicki holds advanced degrees in Leisure Education and Gerontology, Psychology, Theology, and Canon Law. Dr. Sawicki is the administrator of Our Lady of Vilnius Lithuanian Catholic Church in lower Manhattan and Adjunct Professor at Mercy College, Dobbs Ferry, New York.

CHAPTER 15

Interview With Karen Soto, RN, BSN and Rosalee Whyte, RN, BSN: The Challenge of Providing Nursing Care for the Dying

Barbara Stevens Barnum

In this interview, Barbara Stevens Barnum talks with Karen Soto, RN, BSN, staff educator at Calvary Hospital, Bronx, NY, and Rosalee Whyte, RN, BSN, head nurse at Calvary, about care of the dying patient.

> *Interviewer, Barbara Stevens Barnum (BB):* With today's focus on quality of life, nurses are more than ever conscious of how patients and their families are supported during their final days. You two have elected to spend your nursing careers in an institution devoted to dying patients.
>
> I have lots of questions about the nursing challenge, but first our readers might appreciate an orientation to the setting in which you work. Can you give me a brief description of your institution?
>
> Karen Soto (KS): Calvary Hospital, Bronx, New York, is a 200-bed facility that cares exclusively for terminally ill cancer patients. Our care mission is palliation (symptom manage-

Note: Originally published in *Nursing Leadership Forum*, Vol. 2, No. 1, 1996. New York: Springer Publishing Company.

ment), with comfort measures being our number one goal. We really strive to maintain an interdisciplinary environment as well as involving families extensively in every aspect of the patient's care.

We also have a large paraprofessional group that provides a large portion of the physical care, under the direction of the RN. Our cancer care technicians are trained at Calvary for that role, which includes doing dressings, tracheostomy care, suctioning, and other procedures required by many terminal cancer patients. The primary responsibility of the technician is the physical care of the patients.

BB: Many people might expect to find such an institution sad and depressing.

KS: Despite the population with which we deal, Calvary strives to maintain the positive aspects of the patient's life. The attitude of staff is one of caring and compassion, and we preserve a positive approach with our patients and their families, while keeping them informed of what's going on and what changes to expect. Even though it's a difficult time for the families and the patients, we strive to make it as manageable a situation as possible. Usually it's very pleasant. We utilize other disciplines, such as recreation therapy and pastoral care to keep the patients involved in the daily activities of living.

Our environment is devoted to keeping the positive aspects evident. For example, all the patient rooms are individual, and we encourage patients to bring articles from home, to create surroundings familiar to them. All the units also have primary colors. Cleanliness is very, very important to us. Calvary doesn't have an odor like a hospital.

Rosalee Whyte (RW): We have a very supportive environment. Amongst the staff, we encourage people to vent their feelings, to spend time talking about them when needed. We support each other. "You had a bad day today? Tell me about it." I know the person would do the same for me.

BB: Nevertheless, it can't always be easy for staff to cope.

KS: We started a wellness program for the staff. This allows the staff to reenergize, to take a little time out, to relax and focus on something positive, to do stretching exercises, or just have a quiet environment. Guided by either the social workers or pastoral care staff, each session is only about 10 minutes. We encourage nursing staff to be very open about their feelings regarding the patients. We have staff meetings at least once a month or as the need arises. If there's a particularly difficult patient who dies or a patient with whom staff have gotten particularly close to, someone who has been here for a long time, for example, we make a point of meeting with the staff and looking back on how people have dealt with that patient—just to allow them some closure. A lot of the staff do get attached to the patients.

BB: Let me play devil's advocate for a moment. Why would anyone want to work here?

KS: That's the predominant perception, even among other health care workers. Death is an inevitable part of life, and when it's illness related, it can be a very difficult time if the person is in an institution that does not value dying as a unique experience in life. There's only one time that the patient is going to die. For the family, that's the only time they're going to lose their mother, their father, whoever that person is in their lives. If you are the type of person who wants to assist in that experience, you have to be a caring person, someone who is compassionate concerning other people's situations. It goes beyond just empathy. You have to be willing to help, to be available on an emotional level. You have to have a caring attitude in what you do. In other institutions, people may not always be able to do that. Here, there's a real understanding that that's what we do. The fact that we only care for dying patients allows people to develop those human relations skills, to be sensitive to what's going on.

A lot of people come here with a different perception of what this work is all about. That view changes when they actually come here.

BB: I agree that the environment is surprisingly upbeat. How do you keep things that way?

RW: I think we do it by communicating with each other and through the personalities of the people who work here; those things keep it upbeat. Once you come to Calvary, once you've spent 6 months, you definitely want to stay. Most people leave before that if this work isn't for them. The place is cheerful and the people are very courteous. The place grows on you. In other institutions, people are impersonal; here people are personable. That is probably why I have stayed this long.

BB: How long have you been at Calvary?

RW: Seventeen years. The atmosphere is great. Compared to other places, we still have loads of staff to help with care. The ratio of nurses to patients is very good.

BB: Rosalee, what made you personally want to work at Calvary?

RW: I think it was the warmth of the place that attracted me, and that I could give something of myself to these dying patients.

BB: Does that constant giving ever sap you? Do your nurses develop rituals to help them cope?

RW: Not so much rituals. Since I've been working here, our patients are not staying as long as they used to. When I first came here, there were patients who stayed a long time, and you did get very attached to them. Now they're coming in sicker and don't stay that long. The attachment is still there, but not as deep. You still have nurses who will run to the laundry to get a favorite nightgown or jacket, nurses who will try to do a patient's hair nicely. The mourning part: When we see a patient deteriorating, we tend to draw back a bit, not draw back in the sense that we're not in the room, but emotionally. We try to prepare ourselves just as the family prepares themselves to make that separation. In report, we talk about it. We have patients that are suffering a lot, some that are in agony, suffering with decubitus, dying with difficulty. All of us go home and pray a lot. We want their suffering to end. The first person you see the next morning will be asked, "Is so and so still here?" And if they're gone we say, "Thank God." We're happy their suffering is over. Those are the things that we do, some of the ways we prepare ourselves.

BB: Still, I think it must take a special kind of person to work successfully with the dying.

RW: I think I have grown since I've been at Calvary. I came from an acute care hospital, and I love the atmosphere here. I am very comfortable here. I have gone from being an assistant to a patient care coordinator. I've grown in my professional life; I've grown as a nurse. I think Calvary is a great place for people who have a lot of compassion. People who can smile when they walk in that door. I have a family member right now who said, "One day, I felt very down, and you came around and you hugged me. You don't know how that hug made me feel." For myself, I love taking care of these patients. I love the fact that I am able to make a difference. I love the fact that someone says to me, "I can go home and know that my loved one will be taken care of." That's the kind of satisfaction I get from working here.

BB: Calvary has amazed me by its total involvement of the patient's family.

RW: From the day of admission, the families are welcome, at any hour. We make allowances for families with children and for any family members who are working irregular hours. We have 24-hour visiting, so any family member can visit at any time. Even before we had official 24-hour arrangements, the families were always encouraged to visit any time. We have a family room for them to stay over when patients are critical.

On our patients' birthdays, we have a party, with cake and ice cream. Families are encouraged to come. If someone has an anniversary or special day they want to celebrate, we make sure it is incorporated into the day's activities. We make certain that all the families are aware of who's the nurse, who's the doctor, the dietitian, and the social worker. They have a base so they can ask questions. They're given a card so that they know the contact person, so that they don't feel out of place. They're made to feel welcome, especially on that first day of admission.

We also have family conferences on Sunday to help families see that they're not alone, to give them more information, and also for us to find out how they're doing. It's a lot of family contact. Fortunately, we can converse freely. The nurses here are able to tell the families how the patients are doing, where at other hospitals this is not necessarily so.

BB: I know that conferences with families actually take place at Calvary. I've sat in on at least one that included physicians, social workers, dietitians, and nurses.

Since the institution is Roman Catholic, is religion dominant in the care or in patient selection?

RW: No, it isn't. We have patients of all religions; Muslim, Jewish,
and Protestant. Catholicism isn't preached to anyone. Patients
are free to practice whichever religion they choose. The pastoral care is here for their comfort, to meet their spiritual
needs, but no one tries to convert anyone. Religion is not a
criterion for a patient coming here. There's no cut-off point
based on religion.

BB: Is the pastoral care program strictly Roman Catholic?

RW: No, we have two Jewish chaplains and also Protestant min-
isters. And if patients and families want to bring someone in
from the outside, these spiritual leaders are encouraged.

BB: We think of Calvary as a place where patients go to die, but
you also have patients go home.

RW: Yes, we do. Lately we've been sending home a lot of
patients. We have a home care department for continuity.
With our philosophy of nonabandonment, we're still taking
care of the patient, even when he or she is on the outside.

BB: Tell me about that philosophy.

KS: The philosophy of nonabandonment means what it says:
that we will not abandon our patients. If one of our patients
needs to be sent to a nursing home or sent home, we make
sure the facility is safe and decent, that the patient will get
adequate care. We allow the families the opportunity to visit
these facilities and feel comfortable with where their loved
one is being placed. Families are told that if the patient's condition deteriorates or is not being adequately managed they
can return to Calvary; we welcome them any time.

BB: It sounds to me as if you are doing hospice care. How does
this facility differ from a hospice?

RW: Calvary is still an acute care hospital where we are gov-
erned by all the usual regulatory bodies. We still give patients
IVs, and chemotherapy on a limited basis; we put nasogastric
tubes in, give oxygen, administer high-tech pain management.
It's a totally different setting.

BB: I know that at times you use heavy pain control, heavy doses of medication. For nurses on the outside, sometimes that's a problem.

RW: Our philosophy is to make sure the patients are dying in comfort. We do go by guidelines: respirations, level of consciousness. We do have patients that need large doses of narcotics. Often they're walking around on very high doses, 300 mg, 400 mg of morphine that they might get every hour. The nurses who come to work here are asked how they feel about giving large doses of narcotics. We ask because many nurses don't want to give large doses because of addiction. I don't think that's a concern here; the concern is that the patients are comfortable.

We do tell nurses about this at the time of hire, so I don't think we have a problem. If a nurse has a problem with administering high doses, she shouldn't be here. We don't want someone to withhold medication because of his or her beliefs. We look at it in an objective manner.

We also have families that have concern: "They're going to get addicted." We have studies that show addiction is minimal. I've been here for 17 years, and I've never seen a patient get addicted to the medication—you know—where you think they don't have pain and they're asking for narcotics anyway. There have been some who were addicted before they got here.

BB: Some nurses have trouble, not with the notion of addiction, but with death as a side effect of narcotics. Is that a problem for you?

KS: No, it isn't. If you look at it objectively, they probably would die within a short period of time anyway. So the real issue is comfort. That's what you're giving pain medication for, whether it be for breathing, anxiety, or actual pain; even up to the moment of death, they're able to experience pain.

BB: In spite of your positive environment, most of your patients eventually die. One could say that the environment is flooded with death. Do your patients or staff have any experiences related to death apparitions?

RW: Yes, sometimes our patients tell us, "I'm going to die," or that they have seen the light. They'll tell the nurses about the light or say, "I've seen someone calling me." They're very correct. You come in the next morning, and they're gone.

BB: Karen, have you heard of patients seeing death apparitions?

KS: Oh yes, rather often actually. Numerous patients have verbalized that they've seen family members who have died many years ago—their parents or grandparents. I had one patient in particular who said she saw two very large men dressed in white at both sides of her bed. She claimed they were angels and they were just waiting for her. They see people, they hear things; they get a sense of wanting to go home—not to their physical house, but to die. Usually it is those patients who are accepting of death who experience these things. Since these experiences are primarily comforting to the patient, I believe it assists them in preparation for death.

BB: Is it true that many patients experience a moment of clarity, even if they have been unconscious or confused, just before death?

KS: It happens a lot, not necessarily just a patient coming out of a coma. Even patients who are responsive will experience an increase in their level of consciousness. It's when they suddenly begin to talk to their family about things important to them or when an unconscious patient suddenly responds to your request by squeezing your hand. Sometimes it's a day before the death, sometimes a shorter period right before death. Sometimes that's the harder part. Families get hopeful that things are getting better when they see what appears to be an improvement. And you think, "No, everything's not fine." You encourage them to just appreciate the moment. That's one thing you have to emphasize with families: just appreciate the moment when you have it. If they have the patient with them for that 5 minutes, that half hour, I tell the family, "Tell them everything you need to tell them, and they'll hear and understand."

BB: I suspect you see many different patient attitudes and approaches to death.

KS: Some patients fight the experience with every last bit of energy, no matter what their physical situation. Other patients are much more accepting. They know that, not only is death an inevitable part of life, but since they've gone through so much already—so many tests and surgeries—that just living is exhausting for them, a traumatic experience. They can't function in the roles they're accustomed to and that they've worked their whole life for. They prefer not to live anymore. Those patients accept death better than others. The younger the patient, the harder it is. That's not in the normal way of life—to say goodbye to one's children through death. The trauma involved is much greater.

For dying parents who have very small children, it's very difficult, even if they're accepting of death for themselves. The agony of leaving their children behind without a parent is very real for them.

BB: Are there any particular theories that support you in your work?

KS: I find Kübler-Ross to be on target. Sometimes it's not quite as apparent as on paper. You try to put people in categories, but sometimes they vacillate so quickly, it's hard to say, okay, that's why they're doing this. More often, when people are accepting of death, you can look back and see they went through many of the stages.

BB: Kübler-Ross's stages?

KS: A lot of patients go through them such as the denial then bargaining and quite often expressions of anger. Your hope is that they reach acceptance. Sometimes it depends on how they discussed their illness and the extent of it. If they've had more time to intellectualize, it is easier to spot the stages. But, for example, those who found out only 2 weeks ago that they have terminal cancer and have to leave their job—I think they don't have the time to process their emotions. They're just dealing with the shock and the disbelief that it's happening to them. In addition to the patient, each family member is attempting to cope with the situation as well.

BB: Has working with the dying changed your personal beliefs?

KS: It has had a profound influence on my views. I started here when I was 21. At that age, you don't think about death and dying, and it was just a job. My original concept was this isn't going to happen to me; you don't relate to it. But when you get a patient who is 25 or 30 and deal with the circumstances around his or her illness, you learn that you really must appreciate every day and every experience. I don't wait to go on vacation; I try to savor every day. From the more spiritual aspect, I draw on that to help me deal with patients' questions. Working with these patients definitely has brought me to a more spiritual place in my life as well. I find that true for a lot of other staff too. A strong belief I have is that it is not how long I am alive but what I do with the time God has given me.

BB: What is the average age of your staff?

KS: Fortyish for most of the professionals. The paraprofessionals vary more in age with a larger percentage of younger people in that role.

BB: Does the maturity help?

KS: Yes, because they've had a significant amount of experiences in their lives. Most of them are parents and have older parents who have been ill or died—or they have experienced other family members dying. Their view of life is more realistic, and perhaps not so altruistic as younger people tend to be.

BB: In other settings I've seen physicians and sometimes nurses view death as an enemy. You couldn't feel that way and work at Calvary.

KS: That view would hinder your effectiveness and coping in this setting; it's almost contradictory. Especially if you look at what so many patients have already gone through in seeking a cure. You read a patient's medical abstract, someone who has had cancer for 6 years, and you see the surgery, then chemotherapy, and radiation therapy they have endured. They've gone through so much already. There's an arrogance in Western medicine that we can cure everything, that we have the cure-all and the quick fix for every illness. But we don't. Death is a welcome rest and source of comfort for some and we need to be gracious about that inevitable experience we will all have one day.

BB: I know that families can need nursing as much as the patients. How do you deal with that?

KS: In most cases, families need a lot of emotional support, many times more than the patient. They need explanations being reinforced over and over of what's going on, and what we're trying to do. A lot of families don't know what to do. Should they be there? Not be there? That's the time to tell them to just sit with the patient. And anything they need closure with, that's the time to talk. Families sometimes need a lot of working out of their decisions in the past relative to the person's illness. They should have done this test, taken them to this doctor, should have done this or that. We try to help them work that out, that this may have been the end result, no matter what they did. The maybes, would haves, should haves is what many people struggle with. We stress: This is the situation today; this is what we must deal with.

BB: Families must struggle with guilt over some past decisions.
KS: And a lot of anger. We cannot answer for past decisions, but try to encourage them that the best decision for that time and circumstance was probably made.

BB: Do they act out at the staff?
KS: Yes, and you never get used to it, but you try to understand it and refocus their anger. "We understand that this is a terrible time, and it's very difficult, but acting out won't facilitate the process." That's not the way you word it to them, but that's the meaning. You try to break that down a little bit and bring them to the situation they're dealing with now. Usually that anger or guilt comes in the form of excessive demands— every 10 minutes at the desk for something when there really is no reason. They just want some control of the situation.

BB: The situation makes your jobs challenging on all fronts.
RW: The biggest challenge as a manager is satisfying family members, patients, and also staff. You're caught in the middle between things getting done from an administrative point of view and keeping a balance between staff and family. Mine is a very interesting job, a 24-hour-responsibility job, taking care of 25 patients and their families along with 41 staff members. My job starts sometimes at 6 o'clock in the morning, sometimes at 5 a.m. Sometimes it ends at 7 or 9 o'clock at night. But it's always rewarding.

C

Entrepreneur

CHAPTER 16

Interview With Carolyn S. Zagury, MS, RN, CPC: Nurse Entrepreneur and Publisher

Barbara Stevens Barnum

Carolyn S. Zagury, MS, RN, CPC, is founder, president, and owner of Vista Publishing, Inc. She is also cofounder, president, and owner of Professional Healthcare Associates, Inc. She holds a master's degree in Gerontological Services Administration from the New School for Social Research, New York, a bachelor of science degree in Health Services Administration from St. Joseph's College, North Windham, ME, and a nursing diploma from the Ann May School of Nursing at the Jersey Shore Medical Center in Neptune, NJ. Carolyn anticipates completing a PhD in Health Administration from Kennedy-Western University in Cheyenne, WY, in 1999. Carolyn has written for *Alternate Health Practitioner: The Journal of Complementary and Natural Care, Nursing Management, Nursing Spectrum*, and *Revolution: The Journal of Nurse Empowerment*, among others. Her topics have included nurse leadership development, strategic planning, long-term care, grant writing, nurse entrepreneurship, business skills, and publishing. Earlier, she held various positions in nursing and health care, from staff nurse and head nurse, to utilization review coordinator, coordinator of discharge planning, assistant vice

Note: Originally published in *Nursing Leadership Forum*, Vol. 3, No. 2, 1998. New York: Springer Publishing Company.

president for strategic services, and finally vice president of development for a home care company.

Interviewer, Barbara Stevens Barnum (BB): Many of our nurse leaders have taken advantage of today's health care turmoil to try their skills in their own businesses. Typically those businesses have been in providing some sort of health care, consultation, or education. Carolyn S. Zagury has applied her skills in a different way: by becoming a publisher. Yet even this activity has been influenced and even inspired by her nursing. As she told me in this interview, it was the writing skills and creativity of nurse authors that gave Carolyn the idea of forming her own publishing company. Here's how she put it.

Carolyn S. Zagury (CZ): We nurses are talented—we write poetry, fiction, all sorts of things beyond the demands of our professional roles. We're good. I was naive at first—it didn't hit me—you have no idea of the amount of talent nurses have, all kinds of nurses. Before this business, when I'd think of PhD professorial nurse types, I never imagined they could be so creative. My image was that they'd only do scholarship. But we get psychodrama, imaginative fiction, and poetry! Some of the most beautiful works submitted are poetry! Some of the poetry I received from nurses has moved me like no other writing.

BB: I discovered Carolyn and Vista Publishing through a mutual friend, Norma Turini, who had earlier published in *Nursing Leadership Forum.* I have always been interested in nurse entrepreneurs, but now my interest is doubled because one of my fiction books has been accepted for publication by Vista Publishing. Although Carolyn was amazed at the creativity of nurses, on my part, I wondered where nurses like Carolyn get their equally creative business ideas and the acumen and the bold drive to carry through on such risky yet potentially rewarding entrepreneurial ventures. I asked Carolyn how starting a publishing house first occurred to her.

CZ: I got to thinking about a publishing business because a colleague and I had a leadership training manual that needed to be published. I couldn't find a publisher that was interested. Later, after it proved a success in my company, several big publishers wanted to pick it up. Additionally, I had always been a maverick. Although I knew it (the publishing business) would be a risk, still, it was on my mind. Then I was attending a conference in New York City in the Vista Hotel about the time when Desert Storm started. I saw the name: The Vista. That's the name for my publishing company I thought: Vista Publishing.

BB: What was your prior experience in publishing?

CZ: I didn't know a thing about publishing, I had no idea where to begin. I did a lot of reading and talked to a friend. Then I just decided to go ahead and do it. If it didn't work, that would be okay. At least I could say I tried.

BB: Am I right in thinking Vista wasn't your first entrepreneurial effort? You had already founded Professional Healthcare Associates, a company that serves as a consultant to nurse executives and staff. Could we back up and talk about how you came to found that company?

CZ: I went through all the traditional nursing avenues and loved it. Then I went into utilization review. From that job, I developed a tremendous interest in geriatrics. Why, I asked, did we have so many geriatric patients (40–50 at a time in our institution) waiting in the hospital for placement? The answer to that question led us (a physician and me) to develop a renal geriatric program, one of the first in New Jersey. We also created a medical day care program for geriatric patients. We worked with patients whom nobody else would look at. We developed all sorts of programs with nurses, social workers, and the community, scrutinizing and serving all those people who didn't meet the standards for transfer to other facilities. Building appropriate programs for those patients was one of the most wonderful things I ever did.

It also gave me tremendous exposure to the notion of marketing a program. We were successful in attracting funding for geriatric fellows. We finally came in to our administrator with a check for $1.5 million in funding. That's when I learned how loudly money talks. The physician was appointed administrator over a newly created geriatric department.

From there I went into administration, enthusiastic about how marketing could help me achieve my objectives. Then I discovered that the best marketing plan didn't matter if you had no say over your goals. "Just meet my goals, with no vision added, please," was the theme of the hospital administrator. No new ideas were welcome from someone in my role, no changes in quality improvement. I learned that we've forgotten what health care is all about. From my perspective that involves combining business and valuing care. The mentality was bottom line. Get them in, get them out. I guess the best service was obstetrics: you get one in, two out—in and out fast.

I soon had to admit that I wasn't the type to merely implement someone else's objectives. I was disillusioned. It was clear that a nurse administrator was not seen as someone who could go to the top in administration. For my own satisfaction, I constructed a national hospital survey, finding at that time only 12 nurses in top positions, and 8 of them were Catholic nuns. Considering what we nurses have to offer, I was amazed.

Because I saw the glass ceiling for myself in hospital administration, I decided to try a different type of role. I became an assistant vice president for marketing and strategic services. I was older but still the naive nurse. I thought that you could make a difference, but I couldn't do anything. The very first day, the president called me into his office and said, "You may not use your RN."

"But you hired me to bring that nursing background," I protested. For 3 1/2 years we battled back and forth. I could use any title except my RN. About this time a physician colleague said to me, "You know, Carolyn, you're not a team player."

"What do you mean?" I protested. "I'm a great team player."

"You're missing my point," he said. "If you're not on their team, you're going to have a problem."

I went home and thought about it, and he was right. I told my husband, "I want to resign tomorrow."

He said, "Are you sure?"

"I'm sure." That's when I decided to create a consulting firm. That business became Professional Healthcare Associates. I started the business with three other nurses. One dropped out quickly. "I'm single," she said, "I need a guaranteed income." Another dropped out after discovering that business wasn't for her. She liked the idea but not the reality.

Starting a business is hard work, with few guarantees. The third nurse soon developed personal problems, so I ended up owning and managing the business alone.

BB: How did that business lead to your interest in starting a publishing company?

CZ: As I would go around teaching and consulting with various nursing groups, nurses would ask me, "How do I get published? I had to say that I didn't know. And they weren't just interested in clinical manuscripts but also in writing that showed their creative sides. This expressed need led me to the idea of starting a publishing company. Of course, there was still that leadership training manual that needed to be published.

BB: Was that your first published book?

CZ: No, our first book was by an attorney and concerned elder affairs. But on the whole, we concentrated on fiction by nurses. In the beginning that felt like enough without doing clinical materials. Now we're looking at the other side. There's a lot of clinical work the big houses are not publishing. Now we'll do some clinical publication, but it will never outdo the creative works.

BB: I understand that most of your publications are by nurses and that most use nursing, more or less, in their works; for example, novels about fictitious nurses or plots that involve medical knowledge. I know that can't be true for all your publications, because my novel, for example, doesn't involve nursing.

CZ: It's true that nursing experience can be found underlying most of our works, but not all. Also, not all of our authors are nurses, we have works from others in the health care arena. We have published our first novel by a physician. I tell him he's lucky to be with all these nurses.

BB: One thing that attracted me to your press was that you were comfortable with authors who might later go to larger presses.

CZ: We invite authors to use us as a starting point for visibility. We have one nurse author, for example, now on her third book. Nine years ago, no big presses would look at her first book. Then later, her prior publications with us made her interesting to the larger presses. Her third book (at a larger press) got picked up for the movies, for a handsome figure. If we can be a vehicle for the nurse as a creative writer, then we've done our job.

BB: As one of your authors, I know that your business arrangements differ from that of the big houses. Indeed, one could say that your system allows the author to be a bit of an entrepreneur and share in the risk of publishing.

CZ: I'm a small press, so I haven't the fiscal cushion of a larger press. What we do is take all the financial risk of publication costs and then split the profits with the author 50/50. I felt that was fair. If the author has a winning book, the profit will be way above the usual percentage, and if sales are small, I haven't suffered a major loss through high advances not recovered in sales. You never know if a book is going to sell or not. Some have done really well, and there are late bloomers—books that are out there for a while and then sell. One book didn't do anything for 2 years and then took off and sold extremely well.

BB: That's another advantage that you offer an author. Most big presses give a book a very short shelf life and then remainder it. If a book isn't an instant winner, it's gone. Your commitment to keep a book available for a sustained period is an important selling factor from the perspective of an author.

CZ: Yes, we can give a book a much longer life than the large presses.

BB: You must have faced a lot of start-up problems with Vista, especially since you were just finding your way on an unknown turf.

CZ: Yes, we had a lot of problems—exposure, getting relations with large distributors. We've been fortunate in gaining exposure through some of the large website distributors like Amazon.com and recently, Barnes & Noble.

BB: Marketing is always the hardest challenge.

CZ: We were lucky in being able to get in with distributors. Most important, we keep our authors involved with us. They have the final read before publication; they have input on the cover. We also involve them in setting up book signings in book stores. That's very important. Marketing builds on itself. I try to get all our authors involved in visible advertising like this, but not all of them are up to it. The authors that are willing or able to hustle and speak really enhance their sales. I'll even help write the script if an author is nervous about a publicity interview.

Of course, one of the best marketing tools is word of mouth. We rarely do an ad, but we are all over the country at publishing exhibits. Because we're not in competition with the publishers that print clinical nursing books, they don't mind helping us. And we have a website.

BB: I know that at this stage, you are still offering Vista financial support through the aegis of your other entrepreneurial business, Professional Healthcare Associates, Inc.

CZ: Yes, at this stage, every penny of profit out of Vista is plowed back into the business. The other company pays the rent, for example; Vista only pays its 800 number.

BB: Can you give our readers an idea of the sorts of books you have published?

CZ: Many have health-related content. One book, for example, described the journey of a survivor of sexual abuse. I also think of one that was unrelated to health: a murder mystery where a nurse was the victim. I liked the story, so I'd decided to publish it. Others are somewhat related to health, although that may not be true of poetry. For novels, if I love the story line, I'll consider the book. I think that nurses should write outside of nursing, yet it's good to write about what you know. I get very excited about a book that is by nurse but not about nursing. Many novels are that way.

BB: If you were to divide your books into fiction and nonfiction, what are the percentages?

CZ: We probably publish 80% fiction and poetry, with the remaining 20% covering all other categories. We also distribute other nurses' products such as books and audio tapes.

BB: Who makes the decisions concerning what will and will not be published?

CZ: I read everything myself and make the final decision. I have to be committed to a work before we do it. If I'm uncertain. I'll have someone else read it. I'll read it twice. It's probably unacademic, but I have to like a book, and I have to have a sense of its value for the reader.

BB: What do you look for from your writers?

CZ: The work must have something coming from the heart, particularly if it's fiction. The reader must be able to relate to the characters. Are they real? Is the character like the woman next door? One of the drawbacks to getting nurses involved in writing is their fear of guidelines and constraints. I want to give the nurse a chance. I'm not looking for perfect English; we'll take care of that later.

BB: So you will do some book doctoring if it's needed?

CZ: My editors know they must not change the story line. They can make suggestions to the author, but they can't rewrite. My philosophy is give the nurse a chance. Most of us have had the experience of submitting an article and when it comes back edited, it's so different we don't recognize it. Who wrote this article? I won't do that to our authors.

BB: What are your goals for Vista?

CZ: It would be such a wonderful thing if one of our books were made into a movie. That puts your name on the publishing map, and it would be wonderful for the image of nursing. So I look for books that are very visual. When I read, I envision seeing the characters on the screen.

BB: What has given you the greatest sense of achievement as a publisher?

CZ: The fact that I have found a way to say thank you to my profession. We're nurses; that's who we are. I don't want our authors to ever face a job like the one I had where the president wanted to hide my nursing background. It's interesting that an author is a nurse. I want an acknowledgment of that somewhere on every book. It need not be credentials on the cover, but it has to be there. The reality is that I struggle against the discrediting of nurses; I want to put nursing in a more positive light. Showing the breadth and depth of nurses' talents lets me do that.

BB: Can you tell me where you got your spirit?

CZ: I've always wanted to do my own thing. I don't mean this in a negative way, but at first I tried to develop what I saw as a good nursing mentality. I told myself that I should be giving service. I shouldn't be thinking about myself. What could I do anyway?

Then I finally learned and made the break to do what I wanted. Because I had been in nursing 20 years when I started out in business, I had a good network. I got work right away. But like most nurses, I tried to be all things to all people. As each of my original partners left, however, I had to narrow my business to teaching and consulting in special areas—strategic plans for nursing, management in nursing, writing, grant writing—things that are useful and practical and that nurses don't study in their typical education. Then, in traveling around, the idea for publishing came.

BB: On a personal note, how do you manage to run a business and the rest of your life?

CZ: I am extremely fortunate. My husband comes in with me 7 days a week. He has another job, but when he is finished, he joins me. We don't have children to worry about, but I couldn't do it without his support. It's a very difficult trade and a very difficult life to manage and blend. We are committed to the business, but the marriage and family always come first. It's a difficult balance: the publishing business, my consulting business. It's not easy. Sometimes I'm in the office at 5 o'clock in the morning and stay there until midnight. But I wouldn't do it if it weren't fun and if I didn't feel we were accomplishing something. Ever since I was a little kid, I was a maverick, and my family thinks it's neat. My mother doesn't quite understand how what I'm doing is still nursing. She tries to understand. I really believe that sometimes you can make more of a difference from the "outside."

Some people think running your own business is easy. They think, "Gee, you set your own hours." I work more hours now than I ever did as an employee, but I love it. And, if I have a problem, often, I've created it. So I can solve it. We now have published 19 novels, 7 books of poetry, 19 nonfiction books, with 20 more books already in the publishing schedule through the year 2000.

BB: If someone wants your publication list, what should they do?

CZ: Just write to Vista Publishing, 422 Morris Avenue, Suite #1, Long Branch, NJ 07740 for our catalogue, or call our 800 number—1-800-634-2498.

BB: Thank you, Carolyn, you're a wonderful example and inspiration for any nurse who is thinking of trying her own wings as an entrepreneur.

Educator/Administrator

CHAPTER 17

Interview With Marilyn Jaffe-Ruiz, EdD, RN

Sandra B. Lewenson

Interviewer, Sandra Lewenson (SL): I know that you have been at the Lienhard School of Nursing (LSN) at Pace University since 1981. You started as Chairperson of the RN/BS Upper Division Program, moved to the position of Dean of the School, and now serve as the University Provost and Executive Vice President for Academic Affairs. Can you tell me how your appointment to this university-wide position came about?

Marilyn Jaffe-Ruiz (MJR): Thank you, Sandy. I think my appointment is really not such a surprise when you think about my administrative experience prior to coming to Pace. I had worked in nursing service as well as in nursing education, and I always enjoyed it. I seemed to have some ability in administrative and supervisory positions, starting as a head nurse at a relatively young age and then having progressive nursing administrative experience. When I came in as Chairperson of the RN/BS Upper Division Program, in many ways that was the perfect job because I could teach half-time. And I had much opportunity to do scholarship and various kinds of professional activities. I also had a private practice in psychotherapy. But as I started doing more and more of the Chair role and then became acting Dean in 1986, my career took a turn. I focused more on administration and I gave up my practice. I did much less teaching except as a guest lecturer

Note: Originally published in *Nursing Leadership Forum*, Vol. 4, No. 2, 1999. New York: Springer Publishing Company.

on special occasions. In many ways, my experiences and values in nursing have contributed to my having the position that I have currently.

After being dean for about 7 years, I was asked to chair a search to find a new Provost for the University in 1991. And, in fact a new Provost was hired. But, in the process, I realized how much I enjoyed learning about the University as a whole. The opportunity to interact with all the various faculty and administrators throughout the University on all campuses, representing all the schools was very enlightening and informative. Then I had an opportunity to first be Vice Provost, then Vice President for Academic Affairs, and now Provost and Executive Vice President for Academic Affairs. Some people would say that my background in psychiatric nursing was probably the best training for being an administrator.

SL: I would agree. What led you to accept this position?

MJR: I've never been one of those people who set specific career goals and it seemed that new opportunities would appear— I was at the right place at the right time. It is a matter of growing into positions, and having certain skills and interests predominate and others start to recede. I feel that I'm very fortunate that I had so many opportunities to do so many different things. My nursing background prepared me far better than the average person for leadership positions. Nursing gives you the flexibility because you learn so much about human behavior, organization, managing, and interpersonal skills. I think that nursing is an ideal preparation for just about any position. Nursing and education are very similar in that both are about bringing about change and facilitating people to optimize their health and their potential for learning. I see that my role as administrator for health and education is very similar. You are constantly trying to help people maximize their abilities and that's what nursing and education are all about. So I don't see it as very different.

I grew up in a working class family. I wanted to be a nurse when I grew up. My vision of a nurse was a diploma graduate, in a white starched uniform, and doing very much what I saw the nurses of the 1950s doing. That's what I aspired to be.

SL: It sounds like you're happy.

MJR: I am. We spend a lot of time in the administration of the University doing strategic planning, short-term planning, and long-term planning. Just as I was frustrated by nursing care plans, I am frustrated by this, because we fool ourselves into believing that we can structure, order, and control more than we can. I find more and more that we cannot order everything as we might like it and that you need to be as flexible as possible to know what's in the best interest of the person, the system, or the university.

SL: What in your personal or professional background has contributed or added to your role as a leader at Pace University?

MJR: I think that I've a fair amount of compassion for people. I was put in a position in my own family, at a very young age, of being a caretaker. Having dealt with a family disability has made me a humanistic leader and manager. I think that my strength is working with people. My limitations are probably with numbers, and not so much that I can't do numbers but that I don't always trust them.

I think we try to quantify everything and try to make everything bottom line-oriented. One of the areas I had to learn the most about was to understand fully what the business world does. I had to study how the business world operates to understand the operation of the University, to be effective, and to be aware of the bottom line. I think one of my fears is that higher education will go the way of health care. I also know that what has happened had to do with putting a limit on spending. Pace University has a very special niche in the metropolitan area. We serve a population of students who are first-generation college students and they need Pace to get a leg up on the ladder to success. They are extremely motivated and very focused.

SL: How do you balance the different interests of each of the schools in the University?

MJR: I think what I had to learn is that you can't do what you don't have money for. I had to use my skills as a negotiator and conciliator to learn how to do reallocations and to learn how to get people to agree to transfer money from one department or area to another. That is where I've been able to learn the numbers so to speak, and then to use my skills that come more naturally to me, to try to get closure.

SL: How do you see your role in higher education?

MJR: I believe I'm an example of someone who didn't start off in a traditional way in higher education, but that I've done it step, by step, by step, which is similar to what most of our students have done. I think that I've become a spokesperson as a nurse within higher education. For example, I always use the RN after my other credentials. It makes people sort of sit up and take notice, and that has helped me to show them that we in nursing have abilities and skills beyond the stereotypical roles. I have demonstrated that nurses can be valuable contributors and players in the higher education market. I'm an advocate of accessibility to higher education so that a variety of students are assured a successful education. I also believe that diversity plays a big role in terms of preparing the workforce of the future, and that combining my interests in accessibility, diversity, and the value of education have played a large part in my contribution to higher education.

SL: How do you see your role in relationship to your contributions to nursing?

MJR: I don't separate nursing from the rest of the world so much. I make my contributions to nursing by being a nurse. I never stop being a nurse. Some people say you are not a nurse anymore. That's not true, I am still a nurse. I use my understanding of people, my ability to assess and to work with individuals to maximize their health and their abilities. I'm also the resident nurse on the 18th floor where the central administrators and staff are located at Pace University. They come to me daily with their maladies and expect me to know far more than I ever knew, but it gives me a chance to constantly reinforce a positive image of nursing.

SL: How do the other disciplines view your role at the "table"?

MJR: Even here there are faculty members who say you don't have a real doctorate, you don't have a PhD, you only have an EdD and you are a nurse and thus not part of my department or discipline. But once you scratch the surface, what really manifests itself are the insecurities about their own discipline, and sooner or later they recognize my right to be at the table.

SL: You seem very self-assured. You certainly show leadership and have the support of the faculty. When did you know that you belonged at the "table"?

MJR: I often feel that I'm not there. I'm still waiting for someone to tap me on the shoulder and say that they've made a mistake. I'm never confident enough, but my psychiatric nursing background gives me the skills that I need at the table. I think what happened when I came to Pace and began working with colleagues from other disciplines, is that I suddenly realized I had much more in common with other disciplines than I would have ever imagined. When I became a dean, I could see that in my interactions with other deans and the president of the institution. I was getting positive feedback by virtue of the fact that they allowed me to be a chairperson and Dean then vice president. That even if I did not feel I belonged all the time, I realized they could not all make the same mistake over and over again by recognizing my leadership abilities. These were people that I respect and that were important to me. When we hired the former Dean of the Law School, a former congressman, and he first had to report to me, I said, "Oh, my God." I was in awe of him, but I soon realized he acted just like all the other deans. He needed to be supported, and coaxed, and all those things, and I could do that and had a right to do that.

SL: Do you have an explanation for these feelings?

MJR: Interestingly enough, looking at the difference in leadership styles of men and women I think that a man automatically says he can do it, but a woman says she has to learn it all first. Men are more willing to take a position and learn while they are doing, while women want to take the position after they learn it first. I also think that it has to do with coming from a working class background. Those of us who are the first generation to go on to higher education often retain feelings of not being quite good enough all through our lives, contrary to the reality of our success.

SL: Do you have anything else that you would like to share with our readers?

MJR: The whole history of the earlier leaders in nursing and what they faced is of interest to me. There were a lot of questions about gender, in terms of orientation, and what men did and how women are different now. There are so many things to look at, but now there is a variety of acceptable leadership styles. There are people who come in with a sledgehammer, some who are loud, strong, tolerant, or charismatic. We need all kinds. One of the great things about Pace is its size physically and the fact that it allows all kinds of leadership styles. There is a great appreciation and tolerance of each other and our different responsibilities. It is a great place to be.

E

Historian

CHAPTER 18

Interview With
Joan Lynaugh, RN, PhD, FAAN

Sandra B. Lewenson

I met Joan Lynaugh about 12 years ago at one of the annual meetings of the American Association of the History of Nursing (AAHN). Many things impressed me about Joan. First, when she spoke, she made nursing history part of the general conversation, making it alive and real. Second, she traveled to the AAHN meetings with other colleagues and students from the University of Pennsylvania. This group seemed awesome to me because they provided support for each other in their historical research. And third, she encouraged and mentored not only those in her school but others in the organization. By way of this short opening, I want to introduce a leader and mentor who has made significant contributions to nursing knowledge, practice, and education.

Joan Lynaugh, in her career spanning over 40 years, witnessed many changes in the delivery of health care. She pioneered, with others, the nurse practitioner movement, served as faculty member, wrote numerous books, articles, and book chapters, served as editor of *Nursing History Review* and has tremendously influenced the collection and study of nursing history. Joan responded to the changing health care needs of society by recognizing the need to demonstrate nursing's value, the need to expand the nursing role, and the need to pass knowledge on to others. With her insight and vision, she helped to establish the Center for the Study of the History of Nursing at the University of Pennsylvania in 1985. She also participated in

Note: Originally published in *Nursing Leadership Forum*, Vol. 5, No. 1, 2000. New York: Springer Publishing Company.

shaping the American Association of the History of Nursing (AAHN) and has served as this organization's first editor of its journal, *Nursing History Review*. Dr. Lynaugh mentors new historians and practitioners through her many activities and believes that you must be able to prepare the new generation to continue on with the work of nursing. For these reasons, Joan Lynaugh fits the description of a leader, one who is visionary, takes risks, and facilitates growth. For these same reasons, I believe it is important to interview her and share her story with others.

> *Interviewer, Sandra Lewenson (SL):* To start, maybe you can tell us about your background.
>
> Joan Lynaugh (JL): Okay. First of all, I'm from upstate New York. I was born in Canandaigua, about 30 miles south of Rochester. That is in western New York, and I grew up on a dairy farm. I graduated in 1956 from St. Mary's Hospital School of Nursing, which was operated by the Roman Catholic Daughters of Charity of Saint Vincent de Paul, in Rochester. Thank goodness that there was some new money coming in to underwrite nursing education. I was able to get both state and federal scholarship money and went on to the University of Rochester and ultimately earned baccalaureate and master's degrees from there. I worked for about 10 years as a staff nurse and a head nurse in medical nursing and later in intensive care nursing, which was new and thrilling. I had no idea what I was doing, but it was loads of fun. During those years, I finished my bachelor's degree and continued for the master's, which I completed in 1968.
>
> I joined the nursing faculty at the University of Rochester after I got my master's degree at about the same time the school, which was then the Department of Nursing and part of the medical school, was exploring the possibility of becoming a free-standing school of the University. The School was, indeed, created; Loretta Ford became its first Dean in 1972. But in the meantime, in the late 1960s, actually in 1968, Barbara Bates arrived at Rochester. Robert Hoelkleman was already there (Bob Hoelkleman was very involved in the pediatric nursing practitioner movement). Barbara became very interested in the medical nurse practitioner idea. There were several of us on the nursing faculty who were involved and we

were supported by our Chair of Nursing, Eleanor Hall. With Barbara and Bob, Harriet Kitzman and I applied for some of the early federal grants to underwrite nurse practitioner education. That's what I did full time from 1969 to 1975.

It was deeply interesting work. I really enjoyed working with physicians in the western New York area and the very adventurous nurses who were willing to pioneer these new roles in spite of all of the abuse they had to take from their colleagues.

I worked on the Rochester faculty until 1975 when I decided to take a year off and consider what I was going to do next. We had finished all of our grants. I applied for, and was accepted by, a National Endowment for the Humanities Seminar at Ohio State University. The seminar was run by a wonderful man named John Burnham, who was a historian of medicine. I spent part of the summer of 1975 in Columbus and became fascinated with the idea of historical research. I continued with my plans for a year off, traveled around the county, and had a great time, but I never went back to the University of Rochester. Instead, I looked at quite a number of schools and finally went to the University of Kansas where I earned a PhD in American Studies (a combination of American Literature and American History). I completed my dissertation in 1979 and starting looking for jobs having, by this time, spent every cent I had ever saved. It was a lot of fun looking at schools, even though I didn't have any money. Finally, the choice was between the University of Wisconsin at Madison and the University of Pennsylvania. Claire Fagin had become Dean at the University of Pennsylvania and really needed somebody to further develop the nurse practitioner program there. She was willing to support my interest in historical research. She even got historians Charles Rosenberg and Rosemary Stevens to call and encourage me. So, although, I had decided I would never come back East, I joined the Penn faculty in January 1980. The nurse practitioner program, founded in 1975, needed revamping. They were determined to expand those programs and develop midwifery and a move forward with other clinical programs such as gerontology. I did the nurse practitioner work and by 1982, we developed a plan to do some work in history. The faculty was very cooperative and Claire was very supportive. After a lot of deliberation, we finally came up with the idea for the Center for the Study of the History of Nursing, which opened in 1985. My interest there was to find ways to encourage people to do historical research about what nurses do. I wanted the work to be grounded in the very best quality historical research and address the really fascinating questions about nursing that had seemingly were ignored in the past. I was shocked, when I did my dissertation on the history of hospitals, to discover that there was so little written about nurses in hospitals. Amazing!

SL: Can you tell me about your dissertation?

JL: At Kansas, I became interested in the formation of professions and institutions in the 19th century. I did my dissertation on the creation of the community hospitals in Kansas City, Missouri. Kansas City was a post-Civil War city. It developed just as the Civil War was winding down; the railroads bridged the Missouri and Kansas rivers. Kansas City lay right at the juncture and became a rapidly growing city. As it happened, all of the necessary accoutrements of urban life were needed right away. There was a rapid development of hospitals, very much as they had developed in the East, except in a compacted period of time. I was particularly interested in the private hospitals, opened by various religious denominations and ethnic groups as well as in the newly opened public hospitals. In my dissertation I looked at the groups that came together to form the hospitals; the kinds of nursing care that was available; and the interaction between the public and physicians and so forth. It was later, probably after 1985, before I started moving into the 20th century and spent more time looking at the changes in health care after World War II.

SL: Would you say that the two books you recently completed, *Critical Care Nursing: A History* and *American Nursing: From Hospitals to Health Systems,* are in keeping with what you had started in your dissertation?

JL: Yes, at least I thought of it that way. I had gotten very interested in how hospitals more or less captured the American health system. For a variety of reasons Americans, more than other people, chose to focus all of their entrepreneurial, benevolent energies on the hospitals. And, of course, for most of my life, that had seemed like the most natural thing in the world. But then, when you begin to look at what we chose to do, you see that there are other choices we could have made. During that period after World War II, we poured a lot of money into hospital expansion, and what that meant to nursing and to nurses intrigued me. So that's where the little green book came from, *American Nursing*. Barbara Brush, who was a PhD student at the time, worked on that. We work well together; she co-edited *Nurses of All Nations*, a history of the International Council of Nurses, in 1999.

SL: I really enjoyed reading it and I also liked the one you did with Julie Fairman, *Critical Care Nursing: A History.*

JL: The critical care book was fun to do. It was fun to work with Julie (Fairman). We really hit it off and the critical care nurses were great to support us. They gave us complete access to their documents. It was interesting to talk to them, the founders of AACN, and therefore we had a good time doing that book.

SL: What do you feel is your contribution to nursing?

JL: The things that I'm pleased to have done. I really think that the nurse practitioner idea is a fundamentally terrific idea. I think that the work that I did, and many others did in the late 1960s and early 1970s, was useful to patients and very important for nursing and health care in general. It kind of blew the lid off a lot of sort of phony restrictions on nursing practice that had prevailed for 70 years or so, and allowed nurses to do what they already knew how to do. But they really needed both permission and more knowledge to work with patients in a more independent and complete sort of way. We used to say that what nurses needed was more money and a room of their own in which to see the patients. So, that was something that I was really pleased to do. It was a lot of fun, but it was kind of difficult sometimes because there was a lot of stress inside of nursing.

SL: Can you explain?

JL: Yes. Many people in the 1970s felt that it (the nurse practitioner idea) was the wrong thing to do. There were many leaders in nursing who thought that nurse practitioners were selling themselves out to medicine and were actually abandoning nursing. That view was responsible for a lot of conflict.

SL: How did you handle that?

JL: I ignored it mostly.

SL: I need to learn that leadership strategy.

JL: I think what I believed, and I think a lot of people believed, was that those who were concerned about nurses abandoning nursing were wrong, and they would just have to get over it. You couldn't really prove that you weren't abandoning nursing. I mean, you can't prove a negative, so I think most of us just ignored it. We were also getting a lot of positive reinforcement from other segments of nursing, there was a lot of public support and support from states and the federal government, which were pouring money into this expanded activity on the part of nursing. During the 1970s we used to think that health care was a right. Remember?

SL: Yes.

JL: And there was a lot of energy to make that access to health care happen.

SL: That's right, now we just think its managed care.

JL: That's right—only what we can afford.

SL: Now it's a policy.

JL: In the 1970s, the idea that Americans had a right to health care was completely accepted. The next problem was, if everybody had a right to health care, how were we possibly going to give it to them? Nurse practitioners began to address that need and broaden public access to health services.

So, I'm proud of my nurse practitioner practice and teaching, but I must say I really loved what we've been able to do in nursing history. I think that's more surprising in some ways, that is, that it was possible to carve out a place for history in nursing research. Nursing research is so new and so tentative, and people are so concerned about doing it right. Finding history a place in that kind of situation was much easier than I expected it would be.

SL: You can probably document the interest in history by the number of requests that you receive in the Center for the Study of the History of Nursing.

JL: There are many kinds of responses because history is a subject, I think, which must be broad-based. As we thought about developing a history enterprise, we always thought about it as being not just for the most elite, nor as just an 'inside the University' activity. We tried very hard to involve nurses throughout Philadelphia and nurses who had nothing to do with universities, who were alumni of diploma programs and so forth. We also tried to reach out to people interested in the history of women, race, labor, medicine, and so forth. That way we would have a broad constituency for our subject. People have been remarkably responsive to this effort. It was just the right time to do this.

SL: It has made it possible for people to study the series of important nursing collections in one center.

JL: Well, I think we were fortunate. We were able to raise some money. We got into the collecting business mostly because it was impossible to pursue the research agenda without collecting the material. You know, the state of nursing history was so undeveloped, it was like building a house. You had to do all the foundation work because there was so little there, in terms of documents, except what was scattered around in hard to locate places. We are still in the early stages of collecting—but people did respond very well to the whole idea.

SL: In what way?

JL: Well, I think there are several layers. I'll start with the area that I thought would be the greatest difficulty. I really expected more resistance from school of nursing faculty, not just in our school, but in other schools, to history as a legitimate subject for the PhD. Faculty at Penn were incredibly supportive. They never blinked and I thought for sure that they would. Of course, accepting history as a valid subject in nursing research makes everything else legitimate in some sense. Once you can show that these PhD candidates in nursing can do historical research and writing that is competitive in history and in nursing, then you legitimize historical research in nursing. That was one of our main goals. It was to develop a doctoral program and then attract really smart people—the smartest ones we could find. Then let them show and tell basically what history in nursing could be. The other thing that was important was that we have been able to attract money. Those two things, the university faculty support and the tangible support in the form of cash that came from various funding agencies, from people willing to underwrite historical research, and from nurses and doctors and other people who were willing to support historical research, were crucial to the success of the Center.

SL: How do you think that has changed perhaps the landscape of nursing?

JL: It's hard to say. I think that's a terrific question, and as a historian, I probably should quickly say, "I'm too close to it and it is too soon." But, I'll say a couple of things anyway.

SL: I'm hoping!

JL: I think that one of the things that happens as a result of good historical research and writing about nursing is that it changes the landscape by putting events in a much larger perspective. You know, nurses and everyone else are always inclined to just put their noses right up against every problem; we get so close to it we cannot get any sense of what actually is happening. If you can get people to read history, and you can write it in a way they find attractive, then they can see that there is more to this issue than the "here and now" and what they are experiencing. And I think that does change over time. What I'm hoping, at least, is that the study of history changes and improves the way we deal with the everyday issues that are always there. You know, what is the work, who's going to do it, how much are they going to get paid, and does it make any difference anyway? These are kind of simple but profound questions.

SL: Even though we can't really judge the outcome of the long-term effect, I think what you say makes a lot of sense.

JL: Yes, well, people long to know. I don't teach routinely anymore, but I usually do a class or two in Karen's [Buhler-Wilkerson] course where she has mostly sophomores and juniors. I really love to meet with them because they are anxious to know stuff they don't know anything about; that is, the origin of the field or how issues that they encounter now appeared in the past.

SL: It's fun to teach the history.

JL: Yes, it is.

SL: One of the things that I admire about you is that you seem to be a mentor to so many nurse historians, including myself. I'd like to hear your thoughts on mentorship.

JL: Well, it's very enjoyable. I mean, in the first instance, most of us do things with our time because we enjoy them. I would start by saying that working with people who are interested in the same things as you are is a great pleasure. But then the other purpose is that you can't have a movement with just one hand clapping. I mean, you have to have people from every place "get it." If they don't "get it," you're not going to accomplish anything. So we've always tried to be pretty open and to be as helpful as we could and to attend to other people's ideas and plans and all that. Actually Barbara Brodie and I have talked about this a lot. We just don't think that being exclusive is a good idea. It doesn't seem right to say, "I'm doing that so you shouldn't." That seems to be very selfish. So we enjoy the visiting scholars who come in the summertime. We work with various people who want to come and work with us. You always profit by that because they give you new ideas and different perspectives on old ideas. It's been very important to us to do that. I can now do a lot of that by e-mail.

SL: Could you tell me about your participation in the development of the American Association of the History of Nursing and how this coincided with the University of Pennsylvania's Center for the Study of the History of Nursing?

JL: I think the only way to answer that is to tell you the particulars because there's a certain serendipitous quality to this. I didn't know anything about the American Association of the History of Nursing in 1980. I mean, I was in Kansas when it was actually organized; I was writing my dissertation. So I never saw anybody from one end of the day to the next. And then I went to Penn, and I still didn't know anything about the AAHN. But then I went to an American Association of the History of Medicine meeting at Duke, I think it was in 1981 or 1982. I met Barbara Brodie there, whom I knew since our nurse practitioner days. I'm pretty sure it was Barbara who told me about the AAHN. Barbara's school, the University of Virginia, hosted one of the AAHN annual meetings around 1984. (I'm not sure about the dates.) We all went, of course, and that's the best of my recollection of how we got together with AAHN—we being myself, Ellen Baer, and Karen Buhler-Wilkerson. We three were in this history conspiracy at Penn together. Actually I should have mentioned that earlier because it was very important that we were a group. We were a good combination.

SL: You've been together for a long time then.

JL: Yes, a very long time. And Ellen, of course, was very instrumental in moving a lot of these things along. Even though she left Penn quite a while ago, she's still pretty attached to it and so we consider ourselves a working trio or a quintet, I guess. Now Patricia D'Antonio and Julie Fairman are Center associates.

SL: That's nice.

JL: It's nice and it's a lot of support. And I think that is an important element to bear in mind—it's very much like my attitude toward playing together and mentoring. Bringing people together and going along in a direction that's more or less the same—if you can do that, the impact of what you're trying to do is going to be a lot greater and more lasting than if you tried it alone.

SL: You've shared your ideas about the nurse practitioner movement, the Center for the Study of the History of Nursing, mentoring, and the AAHN. What I am interested in now is your leadership as the editor of the AAHN's *Nursing History Review.*

JL: Well, actually the journal was really quite a daring thing for the AAHN to do. There had been conversations, as I'm sure you recall, about having a journal for a long time. People like Vern Bullough, Olga Church, Barbara Brodie, and Rosemary McCarthy, I hope I'm not forgetting anyone, were pretty interested in this idea of having a journal. When Barbara Brodie was AAHN president we began to plan for the journal.

SL: I had just joined about that time.

JL: Barbara really pushed it along. And we just felt we could go ahead. And I had some interest in seeing it through. What made me think that I could do it and might want to do it was my association with Florence Downs, who was editor of *Nursing Research*. (This was in the late 1980s.) Florence was on the Penn faculty, and she invited me to help edit two issues of *Nursing Research* that were historically oriented. One was the 35th anniversary issue and the second was the 40th (I think). Florence was wonderfully helpful in teaching me how to do this. We had always talked a lot about her job as editor of *Nursing Research*, but she also helped by just letting me understand and see how she worked. That experience was a lot of fun for me. I found it was something I liked to do and so when the AAHN decided to take the plunge with the journal, I was interested in being the editor. I had a history colleague, Caroline Hannaway, who was the editor of the Bulletin of the History of Medicine. She is a very skilled person. I kind of copied everything she did.

SL: Would you say she was a mentor or something?

JL: She was a template.

SL: I like that term.

JL: So it was really an adventurous thing for the AAHN to do. And then we made a deal with the University of Pennsylvania Press to publish the *Review*. And that was actually, although we left Penn Press after the first five volumes, very important, because they had very talented people in design and layout, and gave us all sorts of suggestions in terms of how the journal could look.

So, I didn't invent the journal. I took their advice about how it should look. Of course, the most important thing of all was that the scholarship being produced was good quality, and reviewers worked hard to make the journal what it is.

We still accept only half of what comes in, but you know, when you look at the journal, for a relatively small group of scholars it's quite an amazing publication.

SL: It's a wonderful journal. I use it with my students all the time.

JL: I think it is—I think its future is bright.

SL: I'm getting a sense of your leadership style . . . that you are able to motivate people, bring forth your ideas, are willing to take risks, and like to have fun.

JL: I do like to have life be not boring. I think it's a lifelong thing with me. I like to do things that are interesting and maybe just a little bit over the edge.

SL: I can understand that.

JL: Sometimes you get into a bit of trouble that way, but nursing is very generous and so interesting.

SL: Why do you say that?

JL: Generous because you can go off in all sorts of directions. I mean nursing is not narrow. There are a lot of things in nursing you can do and they are all extending. If you think about it, I've gone from medical intensive care, to nurse practitioner in ambulatory care, to educator and nurse historian, and that's only the first 40 years.

SL: You have many more to go.

JL: It's a very big field with a lot of people and a lot of scope and I think it's a great field. I thank God I picked it. I didn't know what I was doing, but I am glad that I did it.

SL: Joan, I really appreciate you having taken the time.

JL: I enjoyed it.

Joan Lynaugh, now Professor Emeritus, is planning to "simplify" her life and will soon pass the editorship of *Nursing History Review* to another nurse historian, Patricia D'Antonio. She will, in the next year, complete her roster of students working on their doctoral dissertations. Her plans for the future include further historical research, noting that she still enjoys reading the people's diaries and letters. She is very interested in how nursing education moved into higher education in the United States and plans to write on this subject.

Throughout her career Joan opened the door for many to study the history of nursing and to be part of its history. She has led others through her own vision, hard work, and great insight. She sees nursing as still evolving and has made us all reflect on ourselves and on nursing. She has contributed significantly to changing the landscape of nursing and health care in society. We are better prepared to enter this century because of her wisdom and her leadership.

Index

Acceptance, in death and dying,
165–167
Accessibility, 198
Accountability
continuous quality improvement
and, 12–13
home health care, 35
importance of, 78
nursing management and, 77
shared vision and, 78–79
unlicensed assistive personnel
(UAP), 114
Accreditation, 7, 144
Acute care
home health care, 33–34, 37–39
in primary care prevention,
105–106
Acute Care Nurse Practitioner
(ACNP)
care planning, 90
coordination of care, 90–91
development of, 89–90, 92
growth in, 94
nursing education, 93, 95
organizational structure and,
93–94
outpatient setting, 91
physician role compared with,
93–94
referral process, 91
roles of, generally, 90–94

specialized procedures, 91
*Standards of Clinical Practice and
Scope of Practice for the Acute Care
Practitioner,* 90, 95
trends in, generally, 93–94
Adelaide Nutting Special Collection,
127
Administration, *see* Nursing adminis-
trators, role of
Advanced practice nurse(s)
case management roles, 8
genetics counseling, 30
Advocacy, 29, 105, 107, 146
Agency for Health Care Policy and
Research (AHCPR), 98
Agency for Healthcare Research
and Quality (AHRQ), 98
AIDS prevention, 99
Alliances, 73
Altruism, 49
American Association of Critical
Care Nurses (AACN), 110, 197
American Association of the History
of Nursing (AAHN), 193,
201–203
American Holistic Nurses
Association (AHNA), Standards
of Holistic Nursing Practice,
41–42, 47
American Nurses Association
(ANA), 24, 98, 125

American Nursing, 197
American Society of Human
    Genetics, 28
Anxiety control, in genetics
    counseling, 25
Autonomy, 25, 58, 77

Baer, Ellen, 202
Balanced Budget Act of 1997 (BBA
    '97), 33
Barnum, Barbara Stevens, 137–147,
    151–169, 173–182
Bates, Barbara, 194
Bayesian analysis, 29
Bedside nurses, 38–39, 92, 109
Belief system, significance of, 47,
    167–168
Biomedicine, 42
Bio-psycho-social-spiritual dimen-
    sions, in holistic care, 41, 45
Board of Regents, 138–145
Bone health, 100
Bottom-up management, 52
Breckenridge, Mary, 104
Brodie, Barbara, 201, 203
Brush, Barbara, 197
Budgets, 77–79, 86, 93, 112
Buhler-Wilkerson, Karen, 201–202
Bullough, Vern, 203
Burnham, John, 195

Calvary Hospital, 159–160
Cancer, *see* Oncology nurses
    detection, 99
    educational interventions, 100
Capitation, 78
Cardiovascular disease, 100
Caregiver burden, 39
Caregivers, interviews with
    Sawicki, Eugene, 151–158
    Soto, Karen, 159–169
    Whyte, Rosalee, 159–169
Care planning, 90, 114
Case management

comprehensive care, importance
    of, 5
development of, 7
outcome evaluation, 8
outcomes of care, 3–5
problems with, 8
success factors, 4–5
Center for the Study of the History
    of Nursing, 196, 199
Change management, 64, 71, 88
Child safety programs, 99
Chronic illness, 37
Church, Olga, 203
CINAHL database, 98
Client goals, 8
Clinical nurse specialists (CNS), 66,
    92, 94
Collaboration, case management
    issues, 3–4
Collaborative care, 58–59, 85–86
Collaborative outcomes analysis, 8
Comfort Theory, 51
Commitment
    in case management, 4
    importance of, 80
Communication skills, importance
    of, 79, 84–87
Community-based care, 33
Complex-care patients, home health
    care and, 39
Computerized nursing care delivery
    systems, *see* Telehealth
Computer technology, impact of,
    58–59, 66. *See also* Telehealth
Confidentiality, 25
Conflict management, 87,
    154–155
Conservation Theory, 51
Consortium of Academic Medical
    Centers, 83
Contemporary issues
    acute care nurse practitioners
        (ACNP), 89–95
    case management, 3–9

continuous quality improvement, 11–20
  genetics counseling, 23–31
  holistic care, 41–53
  home health care, 33–39
  prevention programs, 97–107
  restructuring, 63–75
  shared vision, 77–88
  telehealth, 55–60
  unlicensed personnel, 109–118
Continuing education programs, 26, 95, 155–156
Continuous quality improvement (CQI)
  acceptance of, 15–16
  accountability, 13
  applications of, 12
  clinical efficiency, 15–16
  development of, 11
  effectiveness of, 15
  focus of, 13
  integration, 14
  Plan, Do, Study, and Act (PDSA) cycles, 12, 17–18
  principles of, 16–19
  quality assurance (QA) distinguished from, 11–13
Continuum of care, 37, 73
Counseling, genetics, *see* Genetics counseling
Coordination of care, 90–91
Coronary artery bypass graft (CABG) surgery, 38, 55
Cost-benefit ratio, 25
Cost containment, 65–66
Cost effectiveness, 3
Cost-quality ratio, 8
Craft management, 85
Critical care, 65
Critical Care: A History, 197
Critical pathways, 49
Critical thinking, 38, 65
Cross-functional teams, 18

D'Antonio, Patricia, 202, 204
Death and dying, *see* Soto, Karen, interview with
Death with dignity, 3
Decision-making
  decentralization of, 79
  holistic care and, 52
Delegation, 114. *See also* Unlicensed assistive personnel (UAP)
Diabetes mellitus, 100
Discharge planning, *see* Early discharge; Home health care
Disease
  genetic predisposition, 28. *See also* Genetic counseling
  immunization programs, 98–99, 106
  pathogenesis, 30
  prevention programs, generally, 99
  problem-and-cure approach, 50
Downs, Florence, 203
Downsizing, 63, 71. *See also* Restructuring

Early discharge
  home health care, 37–38
  restructuring issues, 73
Educator/administrator, interview with, *see* Jaffe-Ruiz, Marilyn, interview with
Electronic nursing care delivery system, *see* Telehealth
Emergency care, 37
Employee(s), generally
  involvement, in continuous quality improvement (CQI), 18
  retraining, 17
  training, 17
Entrepreneurs, interview with, *see* Zagury, Carolyn S., interview with
Ethics committee, goal of, 87
Ethics, shared vision, 87
Expectations, 79–80, 153

Fagin, Claire, 195–196
Fairman, Julie, 197, 202
Family, role of
    in home health care, 37–38
    in palliative care, 159–160, 163,
        168–169
Family violence, 100
Flat organizations, 92
Followership, 84–85
Ford, Loretta, 92, 104, 194
Fragmentation, 65
Froelicher, Erika Sivarajan, 98
Frontier Nursing Service, 104
Full time employee (FTE), 78

Galbraith, John Kenneth, 82
Gene expression, epigenetic events,
    29
Gene therapy, 23–24
Genetic counseling
    basic competencies, 24–25
    defined, 24
    purpose of, 24
    technological changes and, 24
Genetic counselors
    education requirements, 29
    role of, 28–29
Genetics Special Interest Group of
    the Oncology Nursing Society,
    31
Gerontological nurses, preventive
    care, 100
Goal-setting, importance of, 78
Grief, stages of, 167

Hale House, 104
Hall, Eleanor, 194
Hannaway, Caroline, 203
Hayden, Carl, 145
Head nurse, 80
Healing, levels of, 156–157
Health care industry, 7
Health care reform, 37
Health policy, 25

Health promotion, 49–50, 104–105
Health status, improvement of, 3
Healthy People 2000, 97–98
Hemophilia, 28
Historian, interview with, *see*
    Lynaugh, Joan, interview with
Hoelkleman, Robert, 194–195
Holism, 50–52. *See also* Holistic care
Holistic care
    American Holistic Nurses
        Association (AHNA), core
        values of, 42–44, 47
    case illustrations, 42, 44–45
    common theme in, 52–53
    decision-making, 52
    healing process and, 47
    historical perspective, 41–42
    home health care and, 34
    models of, 51–52
    nursing interventions, 42, 46
    public trust and, 50–51
    social mission of, 49, 51, 53
    spirituality in, 45, 47
Home care agencies (HCA), 37. *See
    also* Home health care
Home health care, hospital-based
    benefits of, generally, 34–35
    complex-care patients, 39
    cost-quality equation, 39
    cost shift, 37–38
    customer satisfaction with, 35
    goal of, 35
    rehospitalization and, 37–38
    trend in, 33–34
Hospital-at-home, *see* Home health
    care, hospital-based
Hospice care, 164
Human Genome Project, 23
Huntington's disease, 28
Hypertension, 100, 106

Immunization programs, 98–99, 106
Informal leader, 84
Information sharing, 84–85

Information systems, 9, 66
Informed consent, 25
Inheritance, Mendelian patterns of, 29
Institutional review boards, 87
International Society of Nurses in Genetics (ISONG), 31
Interviews
  Jaffe-Ruiz, Marilyn, 185–190
  King, Imogene, 125–135
  Lynaugh, Joan, 193–205
  McGivern, Diane O., 137–147
  Sawicki, Eugene, 151–158
  Soto, Karen, 159–169
  Whyte, Rosalee, 159–169
  Zagury, Carolyn S., 173–182

Jaffe-Ruiz, Marilyn, interview with, 185–190

King, Imogene, interview with, 125–135
Kitzman, Harriet, 195
Knowledge deficit, in genetics counseling, 25
Kubler-Ross, on death and dying, 167

Leadership styles, *see specific interviews*
Length of hospital stay (LOS)
holistic care and, 49
home health care, 34, 37
Lewenson, Sandra B., 185–190, 193–205
Lipid Nurse Task Force, 98
Lynaugh, Joan, interview with, 193–205

McCarthy, Rosemary, 203
McGivern, Diane O., interview with, 137–147
Marketability, long-term, 66–69
Massachusetts General Hospital, 116

Medical model, 49–50
Medicare, 34
Mentoring, 66
Mission statements, 78–79
Molecular genetics, 26, 29
Multidisciplinary teams, 90–91

Narcotic addiction, 165
National Alliance of Nurse Practitioners, 98
National Coalition for Health Professional Education in Genetics (NCHPEG), 31
National Heart, Lung, and Blood Institute (NHLBL), 98
National Immunization Survey, 98
National Institute for Nursing Research (NINR), 31
National Labor Relations Act (NLRA), 110, 115
New graduates, workload and, 78
Nightingale, Florence, 41, 47, 49, 52, 97, 116
Nonabandonment, of dying patients, 164
Nonmaleficence, principle of, 25
Nurse anesthetists, 66
Nurse empowerment, 115
Nurse executives, 67, 74
Nurse managers, 67
Nurse midwives, 66, 106
Nurse practitioners
  acute care, *see* Acute Care Nurse Practitioners (ACNP)
  functions of, generally, 17, 66, 90
  preventive programs, 99–100
Nurse's aide, traditional, 110
Nurses in the Political Arena: The Public Face of Nursing, 125–126, 135
Nurses of All Nations, 197
"Nurse-Patient Relationship" model, 51
Nurse-to-patient ratio, 106

Nursing administrators, role of, 78–79, 87–88
Nursing diagnosis, 52, 105, 116
Nursing education
  acute care focus, 105
  acute care nurse practitioners (ACNP), 93
  advance practice programs, 67–68
  diagnosis, 105
  genetics, 26, 30–31
  graduate degrees, 83, 86–87
  holistic care, 51–52
  King, Imogene, 126–129, 134
  New York University (NYU), 137
  pharmacology, 30
  primary health care, 105
  redesign, 64
  restructuring issues, 65–69
  treatment of disease, 105
Nursing History Review, 193–194, 202–204
Nursing leaders, interviews with, *see* Interviews
Nursing Leadership Forum, 174
Nursing literature
  primary health care, 106
  Vista Publishing, Inc., 173–175, 177–180, 182
Nursing research, 199
Nursing Research, 203
Nursing shortage, 51, 115
Nursing values, telehealth and, *see* Telehealth

Obesity, 100
Occupational health nurses, 100
Oncology nurses, 99
Organizational change, 18
Organizational citizens, 65
Organizational culture, 66
Osteoporosis, 100, 106
Out of the box thinking, 65
Outcomes, generally
  evaluation, 8

  redesign and, 64–65
Outcomes of care, case management and, 3–5, 7

Pace University, Lienhard School of Nursing (LSN), 185–190
Pain management, 164–165
Palliative care, *see* Soto, Karen, interview with
Parenting education, 100
Patient acuity, 106
Patient databases, 9
Patient knowledge
  case knowledge and, 3
  genetics counseling, 24–25, 30
  telehealth, 60
Patient-nurse relationship
  genetics counseling, 25
  home health care, 34
  telehealth, 59
Patient satisfaction
  holistic care, 49–50
  home health care, 35
Pediatric Nurse Practitioner Programs, 104
Peer review, 42
Physician(s), generally
  acute care nurse practitioners compared with, 93–94
  education, 4
Physician monitoring service, 117
Plan, Do Study, and Act (PDSA) cycles, 12, 17–18
Population genetics, 29
Pressure sores, 73–74
Prevention, in case management, 3
Preventive care, *see* Primary prevention interventions; Secondary prevention interventions
  adult nurse practitioners, 99–100
  community-level, 98, 104–105
  gerontological nurses, 100
  immunization programs, 98–99, 106

importance of, 74
individual-level, 98
information resources, 98
occupational health nurses, 100
oncology nurses, 99
public health nurses (PHNs),
98–100, 104
types of, 97
women's health nurses, 99–100
Primary health care
educational programs, 107
nursing literature, 106
principles of, 104, 106
Primary nursing, 92
Primary prevention interventions
integration in nursing practice,
105
nursing role in, 98–100
types of, 97
Priorities, recognition of, 87
Privacy issues, genetics counseling,
25
Professional Healthcare Associates,
176, 179
Project management, 67
Provider knowledge
case management, 3–4
genetics counseling, 24
Psychodrama, 174
Psychological equilibrium, 3
Public health nurses (PHNs)
disease trends, surveillance and
monitoring, 98
historical perspective, 104
trend in, 97–98
violence prevention programs,
100
Public officials, interviews with
King, Imogene, 125–135
McGivern, Diane O., 137–147

Quality assurance (QA)
defined, 11
continuous quality improvement

(CQI) compared with, 12–13
focus of, 12
Quality care, 115
Quality of care, 37, 58, 118
Quality of life, 25, 159

Rapport, 59–60
Referrals, 24, 56, 91
Registered nurses (RNs)
genetics counseling, 29
graduate degrees, 83
as managers, 110, 114
Regulatory agencies
case management, 7
quality assurance and, 11–12
Rehabilitation, 73–74
Rehospitalization, 37
Reimbursement patterns, 105–106
Relationships, *see* Patient-nurse relationship
Responsibility
assumption of, 78
in case management, 3
continuous quality improvement
(CQI), 13
in home health care, 38
Restructuring
change management, 64, 71
cost management, 65–66, 73
epidemiological methods, 73–75
impact of, 63, 71–72
marketability issues, 66–69
nurse educators, role of, 68
nursing curricula, 66–69
outcome improvement, 72–73
prevention programs, 74
redesign and, 63–65, 69, 71, 75
skills development, 66–67, 72
unlicensed personnel, 111
Richards, Linda, 116
Risk detection, in genetics counseling, 25

Salary issues, 110, 112

Sawicki, Eugene, interview with, 151–158
Seamless health care environment, 65, 85
Secondary prevention interventions
  nursing role in, 98–100
  types of, 97
Self-care, 35, 50, 58–59
Self-responsibility, 42
Shared governance, 66–67
Shared vision
  collaboration, 86–87
  commitment and, 80
  educational perspectives, 86–88
  follower, role of, 83–85
  goal-setting, 78
  importance of, 80
  interdisciplinary perspectives, 85–86
  mission statements, 78–79
  needs and concerns, attention to, 82–83
  open communications, importance of, 79, 83–87
  staff development, 80
  values, 79
Sickle cell disease, 28
Silver, Henry, 91
Skilled nursing facilities (SNF), 37, 39
Smith, Dr. Suzanne, 3
Social responsiveness, 3
Soto, Karen, interview with, 159–169
Specialized procedures, 91
Specialty nurses, 30–31, 87
Spirituality, generally
  in holistic care, 45, 47
  in nursing, 153–154
Staff development, 80
Staff nurse
  autonomy and, 77
  restructuring and, 66–67
Standards of Clinical Practice and Scope of Practice for the Acute Care

Practitioner, 90
Standards of practice, 24
Stress, dealing with, 111
Stroke, 100
Substance use prevention programs, 99
Supervision, 113, 115. *See also* Unlicensed assistive personnel (UAP)
Syndrome X, 100
Systemic outcomes analysis, 8

Teamwork, *see* Multidisplinary teams
Technical skills, development of, 91
Technologic-humanistic dualistic philosophy, 58
Telehealth
  benefits of, 56–57
  defined, 55
  growth in, 55
  information resources, types of, 56
  language barriers, 55–56
  nurse's role in, generally, 60
  referrals, 56
  tailored care, 56–57, 59
Therapeutic plans of care, 90
Thomistic-Aristotelian philosophy, 156
Traditional nursing care, 89–90
Trust development
  in holistic care, 50–51
  telehealth and, 59–60
Turini, Norma, 174

United Nations for the International Catholic Nurses, 158
U.S. Department of Health and Human Services, Public Health Service, 97
University of Rochester, 194–195
Unlicensed assistive personnel (UAP)
  arguments against, 112

cost savings, 110, 112, 117
defined, 68, 92, 109
effective use of, 112, 115
historical perspective, 116
quality of care, 115–116
roles of, 114, 116
salary issues, 110, 112
task criteria, 110–111
as threat, 114, 116–117
Unlicensed personnel, *see*
Unlicensed assistive personnel
(UAP)

Value-added services, 65
Values, organizational, 85. *See also*
Shared vision

Visionary leadership, *see* Lynaugh,
Joan, interview with
Vista Publishing, Inc., establishment
of, 173–175, 177–180

Wald, Lillian, 104
Well-being, 56
Well-child care, 99
Whyte, Rosalee, interview with,
159–169
Women's health nurses, 99–100
World Health Organization (WHO),
104

Zagury, Carolyn S., interview with,
173–182